Quick Reference to Common Laboratory and Diagnostic Tests

Frances Talaska Fischbach, RN, BSN, MSN

Associate Clinical Professor of Nursing
Department of Health Restoration
School of Nursing
University of Wisconsin-Milwaukee
Milwaukee, Wisconsin

J. B. Lippincott Company
Philadelphia

Acquisitions Editor: Diane Schweisguth
Coordinating Editorial Assistant: Sarah L. Andrus
Production Editor: Virginia Barishek
Indexer: Maria Coughlin
Interior Designer: Berliner, Inc.
Cover Designer: Tom Jackson
Production: Berliner, Inc.
Printer/Binder: R. R. Donnelley & Sons Company/Crawfordsville

6 5 4 3 2 1

Library of Congress Cataloging-in-Publication Data

Quick reference to common laboratory and diagnostic tests / [edited
    by] Frances Talaska Fischbach ; with 12 contributors.
        p. cm.
    Includes bibliographical references and index.
    ISBN 0-397-55147-9
    1. Diagnosis, Laboratory—Handbooks, manuals, etc. 2. Nursing
—Handbooks, manuals, etc. I. Fischbach, Frances Talaska.
    [DNLM: 1. Diagnostic Tests, Routine—handbooks. 2. Diagnostic
Tests, Routine—nurses' instruction. 3. Diagnosis, Laboratory
—handbooks. 4. Diagnosis, Laboratory—nurses' instruction.   QY 39
1995]
RT48.5.Q85 1995
616.07'5—dc20
DNLM/DLC
for Library of Congress   94-16165
                                                                     CIP

This book is printed on acid-free paper.

Any procedure or practice described in this book should be applied by the
health care practitioner under appropriate supervision in accordance with professional standards of care used with regard to the unique circumstances that
apply in each practice situation. Care has been taken to confirm the accuracy of
information presented and to describe generally accepted practices. However,
the authors, editors, and publisher cannot accept any responsibility for errors or
omissions or for any consequences from application of the information in this
book and make no warranty, express or implied, with respect to the contents of
the book.

Every effort has been made to ensure drug selections and dosages are in accordance with current recommendations and practice. Because of ongoing research,
changes in government regulations, and the constant flow of information on
drug therapy, reactions, and interactions, the reader is cautioned to check the
package insert for each drug for the indications, dosages, warnings, and precautions, particularly if the drug is new or infrequently used.

For my dear ones and my darlings,
Jack, Frances J., Michael, Mary, Paul, and Margaret,
Christopher, Matthew, Joseph, Michael, Michael Jonathon,
Bennett, Samantha, Dick, Ann, Teri, and Juke.

·····················
Contributors

CORRINNE STRANDELL, RN, BSN, MSN, PHD
Nursing Research and
Educational Specialist
Independent Home Care Provider
West Allis, WI

BERNICE GESTAUT DEBOER, RN, BSN, CPAR
Post Anesthesia
Nurse Specialist
St. Joseph's Hospital
Milwaukee, WI

BARBARA BARRON, MT (ASCP)
Supervisor of Diagnostic Immunology
Clement Zablocki VA Medical Center
Milwaukee, WI

JAMES COOPER, RN, BSN, MSN
Director of Infection Control
Clement Zablocki VA Medical Center
Milwaukee, WI

MARSHALL B. DUNNING, BS, MS, PHD
Associate Professor of Medicine
Department of Medicine
Division of Pulmonary and Critical Care
Medical College of Wisconsin
Milwaukee, WI

EMMA FELDER, RN, BSN, MSN, PHD
Professor of Nursing
University of Wisconsin-Milwaukee
Milwaukee, WI

ANN SHAFRANSKI FISCHBACH, RN, BSN
Occupational Health Nurse
Milwaukee, WI

RICHARD NUCCIO, BA, MA, MBA, CNMT, RT (ASCP)
Nuclear Clinical Educator
General Electric Medical Systems
Milwaukee, WI

TIMOTHY PHILIPP, RN, BSN, MSN, PhD
Research Consultant
Chicago, IL

PATRICIA POMOHAC, MT (ASCP)
Supervisor, Immunology
Department of Pathology
Milwaukee County Medical Complex
Milwaukee, WI

MARY PAT HAAS SCHMIDT, BS, MT (ASCP)
Manager of Laboratory Services
Elm Grove Medical Associates
Milwaukee, WI

JEAN SCHULTZ, BS, RT, RDMS
Director of Ultrasound and Radiology Education
St. Luke's Medical Center
Milwaukee, WI

··········
Preface

This handbook provides the nurse, the student, and the allied
health care giver with a quick reference for common laboratory
tests and diagnostic procedures. Chapter One focuses on
nursing responsibilities and presents a model for applying the
nursing process to patient care during diagnostic evaluation
and testing. Nursing standards and protocols for collecting
blood, urine, and stool specimens are addressed in Chapter 2.
Chapter 3 alphabetically lists body fluid tests, imaging procedures, and special studies. Criteria for test selection include
tests most widely ordered, together with those procedures
nurses frequently perform or assist with. Potential risks and
complications mandate that information regarding adherence
to proper test protocols and intratest collaboration among those
persons involved in the diagnostic and testing process be a significant part of the information set forth. The title of each test
includes both common and alternate names, abbreviations,
specimen sources, and types of procedures. The titles of combined tests (such as liver function tests) also include names of
all substances measured. Each test listed describes the purpose
and the indications for the test, the actual procedure, the
method of specimen collection, the expected outcomes, outcome deviations, and abnormal findings and disease patterns.
Interfering factors that produce false test results are also listed
where appropriate.

In describing the nursing role, several relevant nursing
diagnoses are listed for each test or procedure. Nursing activities are categorized into pretest care, intratest care, and posttest care. Clinical alerts signal special nursing cautions. Appendices list standards for critical and panic values (including drug
monitoring), universal precautions, latex allergy precautions,
timed urine collection and handling, and contrast media precautions. Condensed but comprehensive reference sources list
current articles and books that direct the reader to information
that includes and goes beyond the scope of this book.

My hope is that *Quick Reference to Common Laboratory and Diagnostic Tests* will help both practicing nurses and students to provide safe, effective care in the pretest, intratest, and posttest phases of diagnostic testing within the framework and context of the nursing process. If these words and ideas help students and professional nursing practitioners to visualize their unique caring role during diagnostic evaluation, if they help nurses meet standards and requirements to achieve proper test results and patient outcomes, and if they provide a unifying practice model for nursing judgment and activities during diagnostic care, then I will have achieved what I set out to accomplish.

Frances Talaska Fischbach
RN, BSN, MSN

························

Acknowledgments

I want to express my sincere appreciation to my husband Jack who did much of the research for this book, helped with all aspects of the book's development and completion, as well as setting up a wonderful filing system; to Teresa Giersch Fischbach for her dedication to the book, and who took charge of information management and communicated with our contributors so efficiently; to Margaret Fischbach, who relieved me of many worries and consulted regarding the computer set-up of the book and assisted in the typing and preparing of the manuscript; special honor to Kathie Gordon who did a superb job of typing the book, and for her many other helpful secretarial services; and to Ann Shafranski Fischbach, whose contribution and loyalty to the project meant so much.

Mere words cannot express my heartfelt thanks to Corrinne Strandell and Bernice DeBoer, who helped with the manuscript from start to finish. Their expertise and ideas contributed greatly to the format and content of the book. Special recognition is due to all the contributors whose accomplished work makes this book a reality.

Thanks to Dolaine Genthe, Mary Green, Pat Haslbeck, Mary Fischbach Johnson, Frances Nezworski Talaska, and Julie Burgerino for their encouragement and inspiration. Appreciation also goes to the librarians at Murphy Medical Library and Todd Wehr Libraries at the Medical College of Wisconsin and the librarians at Marquette University for their help in gathering relevant background information.

I appreciate very much the encouragement and tenacity of Diana Intenzo in getting this project started, the support and expertise of Diane Schweisguth in developing and designing the book with its special content for nurses, and to Sarah Andrus who helped me persevere and make the experience so rewarding.

Thanks to all.

Frances Talaska Fischbach
RN, BSN, MSN

Contents

1

•••••••••••••

The Nurse's Role in Diagnostic Testing

THE NURSE'S ROLE

Nursing Practice Standard

The nurse supports patients, communicates effectively, follows standards and applies the nursing process model to all phases of testing.

Overview of Nursing Responsibilities

As an integrated part of their practice, professional nurses have long supported patients and their families to meet the demands and challenges incumbent in diagnostic testing. Nursing responsibilities extend to all three phases of this testing process—the pretest, the intratest, and the posttest periods. Each phase requires its own set of guidelines to be followed. Inherent is the need for the nurse to apply the nursing process as an integral and on-going care-giving activity. The nursing process is the *nursing* frame of reference for the medical health care model of diagnosis and treatment. (See Figure 1–1 of nurse's role in diagnostic testing.)

Assessment focuses upon procuring a detailed data base about the patient to facilitate testing and to assure accurate outcomes. *Nursing diagnosis* is a statement that identifies the human response to an actual or potential health problem. Its uniqueness lies in the fact that it is nurse-identified and nurse-

Frances Talaska Fischbach: QUICK REFERENCE TO COMMON LABORATORY AND DIAGNOSTIC TESTS. ©1995 J.B. Lippincott Company

---

Figure 1–1

Nurse's Role in Diagnostic Testing

- Support Patients
- Apply Nursing Process
- Communicate Effectively
- Follow Standards

---

treated. Nursing diagnoses are derived from analysis of data collected during assessment. *Planning* flows from the nursing diagnosis and focuses upon physiological, psychosocial, emotional, and spiritual needs of the patient and family. Care priorities with measurable short- and long-term goals are validated during planning. Age and developmental stage, the setting in which testing takes place, information needs, coping style, and cultural diversification must be considered. Because preparation for testing is often done at home or in a non–acute-care setting, and many tests and procedures themselves are outpatient-based, care planning becomes vital if the best outcomes are to be achieved.

Implementation addresses the actual work and process of executing the plans for the pretest, intratest, and posttest phases. Specific measurable nursing interventions and patient activities are directed toward meeting the goals set forth in the plan. Emphasis is placed upon specimen collection, education, proper preparation, comfort, support, safety, infection control, and prevention of complications. Finally, *evaluation* provides data about interpretation of test results, if goals were met or not met, effectiveness of care and patient status. Whether to continue with, adjust, or discontinue each plan component is decided in this stage. Comparing actual and expected outcomes, along with initiation of posttest activities, comprise the major evaluation components of the diagnostic phase.

At the heart and core of care-giving is the ability to communicate effectively. To apply the nursing process to the care of patients undergoing testing procedures, certain fundamental concepts and ways of communicating with others are key to the success of these endeavors. Education encompasses gathering and dispersing information as well as influencing behavior. In the existing health care environment, nurses are continually challenged to provide detailed information and to teach patients complex skills within compressed time frames.

Children, adolescents, and older, frail adults should be approached differently than the average adult. The growth and developmental stages, as well as the cognitive levels of the individuals, must be considered. Children, adolescents, or adults may have heard "horror stories" from peers. Preconceived perceptions frequently influence reactions to the total experience. Honesty, easily understood explanations, nurturance, active participation, and respect for identity and body image are things that must be addressed with all patients. Because it is paramount to effective communication, the importance of "listening well" cannot be overemphasized.

The cardinal rule for communicating with and educating patients and families is to recognize at all times that the patient is the integration of distinct physiological, psychosocial, emotional, and spiritual aspects that unite to make this person a unique, holistic, human being. It is in this setting, then, that the use of the nursing process enables the nurse to better discern those characteristics that define each patient's desire and needs for care during diagnostic evaluation.

The nursing role is based upon standards. These standards influence and govern nursing responsibilities and practice. The American Nurses' Association (ANA) code, Joint Commission on Accreditation of Health Care (JCAHC) nursing practice and patient education standards, Occupational Health and Safety Act (OSHA) standards, universal precautions prescribed by Centers for Disease Control and Prevention (CDC), together with agency and institutional policies and procedures, are examples of standards nurses are held to. (See Charting: 1–1: Standards for Diagnostic Tests. See appendices for specific standards.)

The specific nursing role functions—communicator, patient advocate, patient educator, clinical collaborator, case manager, collector of specimens, participant in diagnostic procedures, risk manager, partner in quality improvement, and discharge planner—are incorporated into the following guidelines for using the nursing process as the model for effective care. (See Figure 1–2.)

Chart 1-1
Standards for Diagnostic Testing

Source of Standards	Standard	Applications to Testing
ANA standards of nursing practice	The collection of data about the health status of the patient is systematic. The data are accessed, communicated and recorded.	Recorded results of PPD tuberculin skin test reveals a positive outcome necessitating the need for a follow-up chest X-ray. The physician and patient are notified.
JCAHO nursing practice requirements	Patients receive nursing care based on a documented assessment of their needs. The patient has the right to the information necessary to enable him/her to make treatment decisions that reflect his/her needs.	Patient with inadequate insurance expresses concern that CAT scan is too costly. Nurse provides explanation of the indication and benefits of the testing procedure.
JCAHO patient education requirements	Patients are provided with appropriate patient education that can enhance their knowledge, skills, and those behaviors necessary to fully benefit from health care interventions.	Nurse follows a documented patient teaching plan. Patient is provided with a verbal and written explanation of self-collection of clean catch urine specimen. Patient is able to repeat steps of the procedure.
OSHA standards	Nurses keep records of pulmonary function, laboratory and x-ray results, hearing	Recorded results of pulmonary function tests reveal restrictive pulmonary disease.

| Individual agency and institution policies and procedures and quality criteria | and vision testing outcomes as part of a health and safety data base. | Patient is advised to return for follow-up results with occupational health physicians. |
| | Policy statement regarding collection of specimens. Procedure statement for monitoring patient after an invasive diagnostic procedure. | Nurse wears gloves when handling all body fluid specimens. Nurse monitors and records vital signs for specific times before and after completion of procedure. |

Figure 1–2

A Nursing Process Model for Pre-, Intra-, and Posttest Care

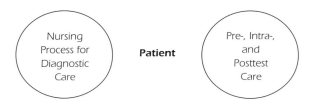

Nursing Process for Diagnostic Care

Patient

Pre-, Intra-, and Posttest Care

Specific Components of Nursing Process

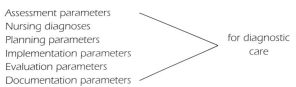

Assessment parameters
Nursing diagnoses
Planning parameters
Implementation parameters
Evaluation parameters
Documentation parameters

for diagnostic care

Pre-, Intra- and Posttesting

Specific Nursing Process Components Applied to Pre-, Intra- and Posttest Care

PRETEST	INTRATEST	POSTTEST
Assess indications	Use universal precautions	Evaluate outcomes
Interferences and contraindications	Collect specimens	Assess compliance
Develop nursing diagnosis	Perform procedures	React to critical values
Prepare and educate patient	Provide reassurance	Modify nursing diagnosis
Use standards and precautions	Prevent complications	Monitor for complications
	Communicate and collaborate	Follow standards
		Provide support for unexpected outcomes

This model provides specific guidelines for the nursing role in all phases of testing within the framework of the nursing process.

APPLICATION OF NURSING PROCESS MODEL TO PRE-, INTRA-, AND POSTTEST CARE

Assessment Parameters

Assess Indications for Testing

- Screen for risk factors or occult diseases
- Evaluate signs and symptoms requiring medical diagnosis
- Rule out presence of disease
- Differentiate one pathological condition from another
- Monitor response to therapy and evaluate prognosis
- Determine disease severity

Assess Factors That Interfere With Test Outcomes

- Certain medications, over-the-counter drugs, vitamins, iron preparations, pretest diet, or fluid intake
- Undisclosed drug, smoking, and alcohol use
- Stress, high anxiety levels, fear, and confusion
- Improper specimen collection
- Strenuous exercise, age, and gender
- Communication errors (improper labeling and incomplete identification of specimen)
- Nondisease factors (pregnancy)
- Past illness and present health status

Assess for Contraindications to Testing

- Pre-existing conditions (ex: diabetes, pregnancy)
- Inability to comprehend and follow directions, to physically cooperate with testing; disorientation
- Allergies to contrast substances (iodine), drugs, and latex)
- Influence of previous testing procedures
- Presence of bleeding disorders

Focus Data Collection Upon These Points

- Age and developmental stage
- Pertinent health history data: allergies, medication history, vision, hearing, and mobility deficits; social history and habits (drugs, smoking, and alcohol)
- Ability to follow instructions and cooperate in procedural protocols (ex: anxiety, mental confusion, physical weakness, casts, immobilization, and diseases)
- Cultural differences and language barriers

- Nutritional status (ex: special nutritive requirements—tube feeding, gastrostomy tubes, IV lines)
- Patient need for information (level of understanding; knowledge of condition, tests, and procedures)

Nursing Diagnoses

Formulate Appropriate Nursing Diagnoses Based Upon Nurse-Identified Need for Care

These diagnoses are also nurse-treated. Suggested examples vary; others are possible.

- Knowledge deficit related to lack of or misinterpretation of information, purpose, preparation, equipment, and need for patient cooperation.
- Anxiety and/or fear related to lack of knowing (not wanting to know) test outcome results, possible need for further treatment, perception of diagnostic procedures as frightening and environment as uncaring and hostile, fear of equipment.
- Ineffective individual coping related to test outcome results and inability to accept diagnosis of serious disease.
- Powerlessness related to unfamiliar procedures, strange environment, cultural differences.
- Impaired social interactions related to language barrier and lack of an interpreter.
- Anxiety of child related to separation from parents; anxiety of parents related to separation from child.
- High risk for injury related to venipuncture; special preparation (for example, prolonged bowel preparation for a patient who is elderly, frail, chronically ill); risks of the procedure as in cardiac catheterization, radiopharmaceuticals, contrasts, and complications.
- High risk for injury related to limited mobility or decline in physical skills.
- Potential for noncompliance to test protocols related to anxiety, confusion, denial, refusal, or inability to follow instructions.
- Altered family processes related to lengthy and complicated diagnostic test regimens.
- High risk for infection related to arterial, venous, or other invasive lines.

- Impaired adjustment related to denial or nonacceptance of test results/need for life-style changes.
- Knowledge deficit related to significance of test outcome deviation and related life-style change requirements.
- Decisional conflict related to test outcome and need for surgery versus medical treatment and life-style changes.
- Pain related to diagnostic procedure.

Planning Parameters

Include Pre-, Intra-, and Posttest Nursing Orders in the Care Plan

- Take into account age, language, cultural diversity, compliance, understanding, and care setting.
- *Pretest care focus* is on proper patient preparation and individualized patient education.
- *Intratest care focus* is on collection of specimens, comfort and reassurance, administration of ordered analgesics and sedatives, assisting physician during procedure, and monitoring during testing. Express confidence in patient's ability to tolerate procedure to completion. Reassure patient.
- *Posttest care focus* is on follow-up activities, observation, surveillance to prevent complications, and appropriate actions if complications occur. Identification of patient and test outcomes and plans for discharge are part of this nursing process step.
- Incorporate patient's need for information as well as pre- and posttest care (self- or nurse-administered) into plan. Include modalities to help patient cope with the actual diagnostic procedure and test outcomes. Be alert to patients with special needs such as hearing- or sight-impaired patients, ostomy patients, diabetics, the comatose, the confused, children, and the elderly. Develop a plan that allows the patient to maintain dignity and some control over scheduling and participation in the process.

A sample care plan for providing diagnostic test information is presented here. Mr. Jones is a middle-aged male (61 years) with test outcome deviations and identified need for individualized social/cultural specific care. This African-American adult's test results show hyperlipidemia, hyperglycemia, and elevated blood pressure.

Specific Nursing Care Plan for Diagnostic Care

NURSING DIAGNOSIS	EXPECTED OUTCOMES	NURSING INTERVENTION
Knowledge deficit related to lack of information about test outcomes and necessary life-style changes.	Patient is able to describe appropriate life-style changes based upon test outcome.	Provide information and instruction taking into account patient's life-style attitudes, and behaviors.

Triglycerides: 150 mg/dL
Cholesterol: 280 mg/dL
LDL: 160 mg/dL
HDL: 30 mg/dL
BP: 190/150

Potential noncompliance related to disbelief that follow-up treatment is needed without overt signs and symptoms of disease.	Patient accepts rationale for testing and treatment and returns for follow-up tests and care.	Provide support and comfort based upon careful assessment of cultural orientation. Teach patient to take own BP; arrange for meeting with dietitian re: low cholesterol, low sodium diet.

Implementation Parameters

Prepare Patient Properly

- Know certain facts: what type of sample is needed and method of collection—invasive or non-invasive; contrast substance injected or instilled; is the patient required to swallow any contrast substance; need to fast; fluid restrictions; force fluids; medications instilled; length of procedure; is a consent form needed; sedation required?

- Review current and previous test results. The plan of care is developed or changed on the basis of these test results. Know how to sequentially gather diagnostic information from records (review the most recent data first to determine the current patient status; then work backwards to note trends and changes).

Place Special Emphasis Upon Patient Education Activities

- Give accurate and precise instructions according to the patient's level of understanding and condition. Avoid medical jargon. Ascertain communication barriers (cognitive, language).
- Provide both sensory and objective information about the test. Talk about sensations, equipment used, length of procedure, people present.
- Reinforce information about the diagnostic process, time frames, and the patient's role. Use resource people if necessary.

Collect Samples for Testing, Assist With and Carry Out Diagnostic Procedures

- Obtain properly signed, witnessed informed consents for specific diagnostic procedures such as HIV, genetic testing, use of injected pharmaceuticals, and all invasive procedures such as cardiac catheterization and certain x-ray and endoscopic procedures in select settings.
- Follow universal precautions, infection control measures, and sterile techniques as appropriate.
- Provide support. Be a caring, listening presence.
- Alleviate psychological concerns. These can affect reliable test outcomes and the patient's physiological state during testing.
- Recognize anxiety, fear, and other patient responses to undesirable test outcomes. Help patients work through anxiety and depression. Assist patient and family to make lifestyle and self-concept adjustments.

Prevent Complications, Provide Patient Safety, and Manage Risk

- Be aware that the most common complications after invasive procedures are bleeding, infection, respiratory difficulties, and perforation of organs.
- Use special cautions when iodine contrast is to be used or barium has been infused. See Appendix A for standards and precautions for procedures requiring contrast.

Evaluation Parameters

Evaluate the Effectiveness of Care During Diagnostic Treatment

- Evaluate progress toward goal achievement. A goal may simply be that the patient can tolerate the diagnostic procedure to its completion.

Interpret Test Outcomes Correctly

- Reassess interfering factors and patient compliance that may influence test results if test outcomes significantly deviate from normal.
- Report critical values to the physician immediately and take appropriate nursing actions.
- No test is perfect. However, the greater the degree of abnormal test result, the more likely that this outcome deviation is significant or represents a real disorder.

Initiate Posttesting Modalities

- Monitor for complications and incorporate safety precautions.

Reassess, Review, and Revise Care Plans

- When tests are completed, test reports become available, new tests are ordered, patient's condition changes, expected outcomes are met, or unexpected outcomes occur: reassess, review, and revise care plans.
- Emphasize importance of follow-up visits for repeat testing and treatment problems identified through diagnostic evaluation.
- Provide psychosocial support. If patients get "bad news," they may not be good, effective listeners.

Evaluate Patient Outcomes and Counsel Appropriately

- Compare actual outcomes with expected outcomes.

EXPECTED OUTCOMES	UNEXPECTED OUTCOMES
Anticipated outcomes will be achieved.	Some anticipated outcomes may not be achieved. Reasons may be related to specific patient behaviors.
Patients and family should be able to des-	Inability to fully participate in teaching/learning process as evi-

cribe the testing process and purpose and patient should be able to properly perform expected activities.

denced by verbal and nonverbal cues. Inability to properly perform expected activities.

If test outcomes are abnormal, the patient will make appropriate life-style changes.

Noncompliance with test preparation guidelines and post-test recommended life-style changes.

Should complications occur, they will be optimally resolved.

Complications not fully resolved; health state compromised.

Anxiety and fears will be alleviated and will not interfere with testing process.

Unable to collect specimens properly or accurately perform procedure steps because of anxiety or fear. Unable to calm and reassure patient.

Does not develop complications; remains free from injury.

Exhibition of untoward signs and symptoms (for example, allergic response, shock, bleeding, nausea, vomiting, and retention of barium).

With support and comfort, able to cope with test outcomes revealing chronic or life-threatening disease.

Lack of appropriate problem-solving behaviors; uncertainty and/or denial about test outcomes; inability to cope with test outcomes; extreme depression and abnormal patterns of responses; refusal to take control of the situation.

Documentation Parameters

Record All Pre-, Intra- ,and Posttest Care

- Enter appropriate assessment data and note patient concerns and questions that help to define nursing diagnosis and direction for care planning.
- Document specific preparation of patient before procedure.
- Indicate that the preparation, side effects, expected results, and interfering factors have been explained.

- Record medications, treatments, food and fluids, intake status, beginning and end of specimen collection and procedure times, outcomes, and patient condition during all phases of diagnostic care.
- Completely and clearly describe any adverse reactions or complications along with follow-up care and instructions for posttest care and monitoring.
- Record patient's refusal to undergo diagnostic tests. Note the reason for refusal using the patient's own words if possible.
- Record all nursing interventions, specific surveillance measures, and nursing evaluations made during diagnostic testing.

2

: : : : : : : : : : : :

Nursing Standards and Protocols for Specimen Collection

THE NURSE'S ROLE

Nursing Practice Standard

The nurse follows agency protocols for specimen collections and handling, uses universal precautions and sterile techniques, and explains the procedures to the patient/family in appropriate terminology so as to educate, elicit cooperation, and obtain the desired expected outcomes.

Overview of Nursing Responsibilities

The nurse's role varies according to the type of specimen, purpose of test, and the age and sex of patient. The most common specimens collected are blood, urine, and stool. It is important the nurse, patient, and family understand collection requirements for these specimens and perform the procedures properly, including ordering of tests and timely coordination of activities. A thorough understanding of principles, protocols, and standards related to specimen collection will prevent invalid results and injury. Specific guidelines for the nursing role follow.

Assess for Interfering Factors

- Actions that may interfere with accurate test results include: incorrect specimen collection, handling, labeling; wrong preservative or lack of preservative; delayed delivery or improper storage of specimen; incorrect or incomplete

Frances Talaska Fischbach: QUICK REFERENCE TO COMMON LABORATORY AND DIAGNOSTIC TESTS. ©1995 J.B. Lippincott Company

patient preparation; hemolysis of blood; incomplete specimen collection; old specimens.
- Factors that can alter test results include: pretest diet; pregnancy; time of day; age and sex; drug history; plasma volume; past and present illness history/health status; deficient patient knowledge/understanding; position or activity at time specimen was obtained; stress—physical and emotional; noncompliance; postprandial status (time patient last ate); and undisclosed drug or alcohol usage.

Prepare the Patient Properly

This process is crucial for obtaining accurate test results.

- Fasting, special diets, activity restrictions, withholding of selected medications or other special preparation are some components of the pretest phase. When in doubt about holding medication, confer with laboratory staff and patient's physician.
- Isolation precautions should be observed where necessary. For instance, with the TB patient, masks should be worn. Universal precautions are mandatory. In certain instances, sterile procedures may be necessary. For example, contamination of a clean-catch or sterile urine specimen with genital organisms could invalidate test results.

Be Aware of Legal Implications Related to Specimen Collection

- These include the patient's right to information including risks and outcome, properly signed and witnessed consent forms, if required. Testing for drug abuse involves unique problems. A legal chain of custody may be required to protect the specimen. This means that each time the specimen changes hands, the person receiving it becomes the documented holder of the specimen and is responsible for the specimen's integrity. For example, persons being tested for drugs frequently try to invalidate urine screening tests by adding substances, diluting urine, or substituting another person's urine. In order to prevent substitution before collecting such a specimen, it may be necessary to verify the patient's identity by photograph.

Consider Ethical Implications

- Maintaining confidentiality of information is a given. It becomes especially relevant when obtaining specimens for

HIV. Reporting of some infectious diseases to state and federal centers for disease control may be mandatory, even if the patient objects to these actions.

Use Safety Measures

• Patient safety and well-being should be optimized by detecting and/or preventing complications. After testing, the patient's behavior, appearance, response (acceptance or nonacceptance) should be observed and documented. For example, patients with bleeding problems or immune system disorders need to be protected from injury and infection.

Observe Infection Control and Universal Precautions

• In spite of using universal precautions, caregivers have the right to know the diagnosis of the patients they care for so that they can obtain and handle diagnostic specimens properly in order to minimize risks to themselves. Proper protective clothing and devices must be worn, and procurement and disposal of specimens according to OSHA standards must be adhered to. See standards for universal precautions in appendix. Isolation precautions (e.g., enteric, acid-fast bacillus [AFB]) should be used as necessary if associated conditions such as infectious diarrhea or tuberculosis are suspected or diagnosed.

Store and Transport Specimens

• After specimen is collected, it should be stored properly or transported to the laboratory immediately. Failure to do so may result in specimen deterioration. For example, urine pH becomes alkaline due to bacterial growth if the specimen stands more than 30 minutes. Failure to follow protocols leads to repeat testing, increasing costs to patient, institution, and third party payor. "STAT" tests should be hand-carried to laboratory and should be documented as such.

NURSING PROTOCOLS FOR BLOOD SPECIMEN COLLECTION

Blood collection may be obtained through skin puncture (capillary blood), venipuncture, arterial puncture, or bone marrow aspiration. (See Chapter 3 for bone marrow test.) The type of blood sample—whole blood, plasma, or serum—varies with the specific test. Equipment (automated vs. manual system), type of blood sample, collection site, technique, and patient's age and condition determine method of collection.

Blood collection tubes have color-coded stoppers that indicate the type of additives in the tube. The following guide determines specimen collection tube.

COLLECTION CONTAINER	USE
Blue (sodium citrate and citric acid additive)	Plasma—coagulation studies
Black (sodium oxalate additive)	Plasma—certain coagulation studies
Grey (glycolytic inhibitor such as oxalate and fluoride)	Serum and plasma—glucose determinations
Red (no additives)	Serum—chemistry, serology and blood banking
Lavender (EDTA-ethylene diamine-tetra acetic acid)	Whole blood and plasma—hematology, chemistry, and blood banking
Green (heparin additive)	Arterial blood gases and special tests such as ammonia levels, hormones, and electrolytes

Nursing Role

The nurse's role in blood collection will vary according to the type of specimen collected and the patient's condition. Universal precautions must be observed with *all* blood collection procedures including proper disposal of medical wastes.

Skin Puncture (Capillary Blood)

Capillary blood samples require a skin puncture of the fingertip or earlobe of an adult. For children, the tip of the finger is often used. Infants under 1 year of age and neonates yield the best sample from the great toe or heel. The heel or toe may need to be used in adults when veins are sclerosed.

Pretest Care

Explain the procedure and purpose of test to patient or parents to obtain informed consent. A warm, moist compress may be applied to the puncture site for about 10 minutes prior to the procedure to dilate the blood vessels. Assess for interfering factors:

- Inadequate blood supply due to cold, cyanosis, swelling or edema, or ineffective process of collection.
- Blood sample dilution can result from improper squeezing of puncture site area or not wiping off the first drop of blood.
- Red cell morphology—caused by residual alcohol used for site cleansing or inadequate drying prior to puncture.
- Epithelial or endothelial cells caused by using the first drop of blood render count inaccurate.

Intratest Care

- Observe universal precautions.
- Assess puncture site for interfering factors—avoid using the lateral aspect of the heel where the plantar artery is located.
- Disinfect skin using 70% alcohol or Betadine and wipe dry with sterile gauze. Allow Povidone iodine [Betadine] to dry thoroughly for effectiveness.
- Create stasis by pressing on distal joint of finger to produce redness at the tip.
- Puncture the skin sharply, quickly, and deep enough to get a free flow of blood. Discard the first drop of blood.
- After collection, briefly apply pressure and a small, sterile dressing to the puncture site.
- Label the specimen properly, send it to the laboratory promptly, and document pertinent information.

Posttest Care

- The dressing may be removed after a few hours if bleeding has stopped. Occasionally, a small bruise or minimal discomfort may occur.

Venipuncture (Venous Blood)

Most blood studies require venous blood samples. Care must be taken to avoid hemolysis or hemoconcentration of the sample and to prevent hematoma, damage to the veins, infection, and discomfort. The most common venipuncture site is the antecubital fossa. However, the wrist area, forearm, or the dorsum of the hand or foot may be used.

Pretest Care

- Diagnostic blood tests may require dietary restrictions or fasting for 8 to 12 hours pretest. Drugs used should be noted on requisition form or computer screen as they may affect results.

- Warm, moist compresses to the draw site or lowering the arm prior to the procedure may help to distend veins that are difficult to find. Be ready to provide assistance if patient becomes lightheaded or faint.

·············
CLINICAL ALERT

◊ Strenuous activity prior to the draw can alter results. Body fluids shift from the vascular bed to the tissue spaces resulting in hemoconcentration. It may take 20–30 minutes for fluid levels to re-establish equilibrium. Thus, rest and decreased stress prior to blood studies is important.
·············

- Assess for other interfering factors which include hemolysis, cellulitis, phlebitis, venous obstruction, lymphangitis, or arteriovenous fistulas or shunts. To avoid spurious test results from IV solutions, do not draw blood above an intravenous catheter or infusion site. Choose a site distal to the IV site if no other alternative site is available. Hemoconcentration may be caused by leaving the tourniquet on for more than 1 minute.

Intratest Care

- Observe universal precautions.
- Apply a snug tourniquet above puncture site unless veins are very prominent and instruct patient to make a fist several times to further enlarge veins.
- Cleanse and dry puncture site. Disinfect skin using 70% alcohol or Betadine and wipe dry with sterile gauze.
- To keep the vein from moving, draw skin taut over the vein and press below puncture site with the thumb.
- Hold syringe or evacuation tube with the needle bevel up and the shaft parallel to the path of the vein at a 15-degree angle to the vein and gently insert the needle into the vein. If using a syringe, watch for blood in the needle hub and then gently pull back on the plunger to withdraw blood. Transfer the blood into the proper tubes by piercing the stopper with the needle. If using an evacuation tube, look for blood inside the needle holder, then push the evacuation tube onto the needle. Blood will automatically flow into the tube.
- Release the tourniquet as soon as an adequate blood flow has been established. If drawing multiple samples, repeat the procedure.

• After obtaining blood sample, remove needle. Apply gentle pressure and a small, sterile dressing to the area until the bleeding stops.
• Gently invert the collection tubes several times to blend the sample. Do not shake. Check for clots or clumps. If none present, send labelled specimen to the laboratory immediately. Document pertinent information in health care record.

Posttest Care

• Check patient and puncture site; instruct patient to lie down and rest. Watch for signs of anxiety or other complications such as: hematoma, infection (septic phlebitis), or vasovagal syncope.
• Warm compresses may be applied to site for discomfort. If venous bleeding is excessive and persists for longer than 5 minutes, the physician should be notified.

•••••••••••••••
CLINICAL ALERT

◊ Blood samples may be drawn off central lines. A physician's order is normally required. Agency protocols and guidelines must be strictly followed.
•••••••••••••••

Arterial Puncture (Arterial Blood)

Arterial blood samples are necessary for arterial blood gases (ABGs) and are usually performed by a physician or a specially trained nurse or technician because of potential risks inherent in this procedure. They are normally collected directly from the radial, brachial, or femoral arteries. If patient has an arterial line in place (most frequently in the radial artery), samples can be drawn from this line.

Pretest Care

• Assess patient for the following contraindications to an arterial "stick": absence of a palpable radial artery pulse, a positive Allen's test (only one artery supplying blood to the hand); cellulitis around the area of the radial artery; arteriovenous fistula or shunt; severe thrombocytopenia (platelet count <20,000/µL); prolonged prothrombin time or partial thromboplastin time (>1.5 times the control = relative contraindication). A Doppler probe or finger pulse transducer may be used to assess circulation and perfusion in dark-skinned or uncooperative patients.

• Before drawing an arterial blood sample, record the current oxygen therapy, hemoglobin, and temperature. If patient has been recently suctioned or placed on a ventilator, or if oxygen concentrations have been changed, wait at least 15 minutes before drawing the sample. This allows circulating blood levels to return to baseline levels. Hyperthermia and hypothermia also influence oxygen release from hemoglobin at the tissue level.

Intratest Care

• Observe universal precautions and follow agency protocols.
• Extend the upper arm, volar side up, on a stable surface. Palpate the radial artery until a strong pulse is felt. Perform the Allen's test when assessing the radial artery. The femoral artery may be used when neither the brachial or radial artery is an option. Entering the femoral artery presents an increased risk of severe bleeding. The site must be observed conscientiously.
• Place a rolled-up towel under the patient's wrist to hyperextend the wrist if necessary. Area can be anesthetized with a local anesthetic that *does not* contain epinephrine. The epinephrine will cause the vessels to constrict and the puncture may then be difficult, if not impossible. Never make more than two attempts at any single site.
• Cleanse site with an antiseptic solution; dry completely. Using a 20–21 gauge needle and a sterile heparinized syringe, line the needle bevel up; puncture the skin and directly enter the artery at a 45-degree angle for the radial artery, 60-degree angle for the brachial artery, and 90-degree angle for the femoral artery. Advance the needle but don't pull back on the plunger. When the artery is entered, the arterial pressure will push the plunger out as the syringe fills.
• Collect 3–10 mL of blood. Remove the needle and apply firm, continuous pressure with a sterile gauze pad over the site for several minutes. Expel the air from the syringe sample and cap the needle tightly. (Residual air can alter ABG values significantly.) Take labelled sample to lab immediately. If more than a few minutes elapse before lab receives sample, pack the syringe in crushed ice to prevent metabolic changes in the sample. Deliver specimen to lab as soon as possible.
• Maintain firm pressure on puncture site for several minutes to prevent bleeding and hematoma formation. (If patient is on anticoagulation therapy, maintain pressure longer.) After

bleeding stops, apply a firm pressure dressing but do not encircle the entire wrist. Leave this on at least 24 hours. Instruct patient to report any signs of bleeding from the site promptly.
- For patients requiring frequent arterial blood monitoring, an indwelling arterial catheter (line) may be used. Follow agency protocols for obtaining blood samples from the arterial line. Procedures vary between neonates, pediatric, and adult patients. (See Arterial Blood Gas Tests in Chapter 3.)
- Label all specimens appropriately and document pertinent information in the health care record.

Posttest Care

- Posttest assessment should include color, motion, sensation, degree of warmth, capillary refill time, and quality of pulse in the affected extremity.
- Monitor puncture site and dressing closely for arterial bleeding for several hours. Patient should not do any vigorous activity with the extremity for at least 24 hours.

NURSING PROTOCOLS FOR URINE SPECIMEN COLLECTION

Composition of urine changes continuously through the 24-hour period and, because of this, different types of specimens may be ordered. These include: single random specimen, second (double)-voided specimen, timed specimen, pediatric specimen, clean-catch midstream specimen, catheter specimen, first morning specimen, fasting specimen, and suspected substance abuse specimen. Random, second-voided, catheter, and clean-catch midstream specimens can be collected any time, whereas first morning, fasting, or timed specimens require collection at specific times.

Nursing Role

Pretest Care

- Education will vary according to type of urine specimen required and patient's ability to cooperate with specimen collection. Clear instructions and assessment of the patient's understanding of what to expect is the key to a successful outcome.
- Assess for presence of interfering factors which may affect test outcome: patient use of illegal drugs, detergents, sodium

chloride, or blood in urine, strenuous activity (causes proteinuria), time of day (urine is concentrated in the early morning), food consumption (glycosuria increases after meals), and feces, toilet paper, vaginal discharge, blood, or semen contaminate the specimen. Unrefrigerated specimens may undergo composition resulting in changes such as alkalinity, casts, red blood cells, very low or very high pH components. Failure to follow collection instructions, inadequate fluid intake, medication, or certain foods may also interfere with test results.

- Assess patient's usual urinating habits and encourage fluid intake (unless contraindicated). Provide verbal and written directions for self-collection of specimens.

Intratest Care

- Observe universal precautions.
- Specimens should be voided into clean urinals or bedpans or transferred into urine specimen containers and properly sealed. Cleanse outside of receptacle if soiled.
- Examine urine for amount, odor, color, appearance, blood, mucus, or pus. Document observations.
- Label specimens accurately and send them to laboratory promptly or refrigerate. All urine specimens should be sent to lab in the proper container immediately after collection. If there will be a delay, refrigerate specimen.
- Obtain specimen as indicated:

Random collection specimen

- These may be collected any time. Early morning specimens are more concentrated and best for routine urinalysis.
- Provide patient with proper container and appropriate instructions the evening prior to the test.

Second voided specimen

- These specimens provide less concentrated specimens but more accurately reflect the urine components.
- Void and discard first urine specimen, then drink one glass of water to stimulate urine production. Void 30 minutes later into the proper receptacle.

First morning and fasting collections

- Void and discard urine at bed time. For a fasting specimen, restrict food and fluids after midnight.

- Collect first void in morning. Patients who must void during the night should note the time on the specimen label (for example, "Urine specimen, 3:20 AM to 8:00 AM").

Clean catch midstream

- This method is often used for random collection to reduce bacterial counts. The urethral area should be thoroughly cleansed with an antiseptic wash prior to voiding.
- For males, cleanse tip of penis with antiseptic swabs by wiping in circular motion away from the urethra.
- For females, separate labia before cleansing and during collection. Cleanse each side of urinary meatus and down center as the last wipe. Always wipe from front to back.
- Initiate voiding into toilet or bedpan first. Interrupt voiding briefly, then void into a *sterile* collection container, taking care not to contaminate the inner surface or inside portion of the lid of the container.

Pediatric specimens

- For infants, same basic collection procedures are used for all types of specimens. Thoroughly cleanse and dry urethral area with infant in the supine position, hips externally rotated and abducted and knees bent (frog position). Then apply urine collection bag.
- For males, apply the device over penis and scrotum and press flaps of collection bag closely against perineum to ensure a tight fit.
- For females, apply the device to the perineal area, by starting at the point between anus and vagina and working towards pubic area.
- Cover collection bag with a diaper to prevent dislodging. If possible, elevate head of the bed to facilitate drainage into collection bag.

Collection of urine from a catheter

- Follow agency protocols for straight, one-time catheterization. Allow a few milliliters of urine to drain out before collecting the actual specimen into a sterile container. If an indwelling catheter is in place, clamp catheter for 30 minutes prior to collection *unless contraindicated* (bladder surgery). Wipe sample port with an alcohol swab, insert a needle into port, aspirate sample with a syringe, and transfer to a specimen container.

- If catheter is self-sealing rubber (never with silicone or plastic), the process used is the same, except the actual catheter is pierced near the area where it joins the collection bag. (Never insert needle into catheter shaft or into lumen because *the channel for the balloon may be punctured and the balloon will then deflate*.)
- **Be sure to unclamp the catheter after the specimen collection**.

Urine collection for suspected substance abuse

- The actual procurement or delivery of a 50-mL random urine sample needs to be witnessed by a trained/designated individual. This sample is collected and tagged with a numerical code and is placed into a plastic heat-sealed sack marked with a special seal to prevent tampering.
- A "chain of custody" document is originated at time of sample collection. The person who provides the urine specimen signs the document, as does every person who handles the sample thereafter. After both initial and confirmatory testing, the sample is resealed, marked, and securely stored for a minimum of 30 days.

Timed specimen collection

- These specimens are collected over a specific time period over 2–24 hours. Explain procedure carefully and provide written instructions if necessary to patient. **The total specimen must be collected**. If any part of the specimen is lost, entire collection process must start over from the beginning or the results will be inaccurate.
- Emphasize dietary, drug, or activity restrictions. Some of these apply to several days before the test.
- Use appropriate collection container. Some tests may require preservatives or refrigeration of specimen. Label container properly. Include time test begins and ends.
- Signs that say "DO NOT DISCARD URINE" or "SAVE ALL URINE" serve as reminders that the specimen collection is in progress.
- The patient should void immediately before beginning the timed collection. Discard this urine and record this time. From this time forward, collect all urine for the designated time period and transfer it to proper container. *Do not* mix stool or toilet paper with urine. Patient should void and save urine prior to defecating. At the end of the specified time

period, patient should void last collected specimen. This completes the collection process.

Posttest Care

• Use universal precautions when handling specimens. Document type of specimen, test performed, disposition of specimen, color, amount, odor and appearance, and time collected in health care record. Transfer specimens to lab. If unable to do so immediately, refrigerate specimen (unless contraindicated) until transfer can be done.

NURSING PROTOCOLS FOR
STOOL SPECIMEN COLLECTION

Collection of stool for fecal studies is usually a one-time random specimen collection. However, some studies may require more extensive samples as in the case of testing for occult blood or fat. Because the specimen cannot be obtained on demand, it is important to instruct the patient carefully before the test so the specimen is obtained when the opportunity presents itself. Written instructions should reduce confusion about what is necessary.

Nursing Role

Pretest Care

• Explain purpose and procedure for specimen collection. Provide proper containers and other supplies. Use language patient understands. Respect patient's dignity and sensitivity to a potentially embarrassing situation. If possible, barium studies of the GI tract should be done after stool specimens are obtained.

• Assess for interfering factors. Ingesting certain foods (for example, red meat) may alter occult blood test results. Barium sulfate in the GI tract or certain medications (tetracycline, anti-diarrheal agents affect parasite detection) may interfere with accurate results. Certain disease states such as malabsorption syndrome can interfere with test outcomes. Contamination with urine or toilet paper, or not having a representative portion of the entire stool, may lead to inaccurate results. Life-style, personal habits, travel, working and environment, and bathroom accessibility are some of the factors that may interfere with proper sample procurement.

Intratest Care

- Type of stool analysis ordered will determine collection process. Observe universal precautions when handling specimens. Patients need to be instructed in proper hand washing techniques. Provide for and respect patient's privacy.
- Patient should evacuate stool into a clean, dry bedpan or a wide-mouth container. Toilet tissue and urine must not be mixed with stool specimen.
- Signs that say "DO NOT DISCARD STOOL" or "SAVE ALL STOOL" serve as reminders that specimen collection is in progress.
- Transfer first, middle, and last parts of stool to specimen container with a tongue blade. Include blood, pus, mucus, and any other unusual-appearing parts of sample. Dispose of remaining stool and supplies in proper manner.
- Label specimen properly and send sealed container to laboratory immediately. The way the specimen is handled will vary according to the test ordered. For example, a warm specimen is needed for ova and parasite studies.
- Document appropriate information in health care record. Include information about stool appearance and characteristics and test to be performed.

Posttest Care

- Provide patient the opportunity to cleanse hands and perineal area or assist if necessary.

3

❖❖❖❖❖❖❖❖❖❖❖❖

Alphabetical List of Laboratory Tests of Body Fluids, Imaging Procedures, and Special Studies of Body Functions

THE NURSE'S ROLE

Nursing Practice Standard

The nurse knows the purpose, procedure, indications, potential risks, complications, and outcomes. The nurse applies this knowledge and the nursing process to all phases of testing to achieve the proper test results and expected patient outcomes.

Overview of Nursing Responsibilities

Nurses need a specialized knowledge base to provide safe, effective care and to visualize their unique caring role during diagnostic testing. The information provided about each test (as well as guidelines presented in Chapters 1 and 2) is part of this knowledge base.

Tests, Procedures, and Special Studies, A through X

• Please note that some tests have been combined: adrenal function tests, amniotic fluid analysis, antinuclear antibodies, arterial blood gases, blood groups and types, blood glucose tests, cardiac enzymes, coagulation tests, cerebrospinal fluid analysis, cholesterol tests, complete blood count, electrolyte tests, heart scans, immune function tests, iron tests, kidney function tests, liver function tests, pancreatic function

Frances Talaska Fischbach: QUICK REFERENCE TO COMMON LABORATORY AND DIAGNOSTIC TESTS. ©1995 J.B. Lippincott Company

tests, protein, pulmonary function tests, routine urinalysis, skin tests, stool analysis, and thyroid function tests.
- Also note that the title of each test includes both common and alternate names, abbreviations, specimen sources, and types of procedures. The titles of combined tests such as electrolytes also include names of all substances measured: calcium, magnesium, potassium, chloride, and phosphate.

Abdominal Ultrasound— Abdomen Sonogram, Aortic Ultrasound, Upper Abdominal Echogram

Ultrasound Imaging

This noninvasive procedure visualizes all upper abdominal organs including the liver, biliary tract, gall bladder, pancreas, kidneys, spleen, and abdominal aorta and its major branches.

Indications

- Evaluate and characterize abdominal pathologies associated with abdominal pain, increased abdominal girth, generalized ill health, weight loss and/or fever.
- Characterize known or suspected masses and determine cause of jaundice.
- Screen for abdominal aortic aneurysms and stage known carcinomas.
- Guidance during biopsy, cyst aspiration, and other invasive procedures.

Expected Test Outcomes

Normal sonographic anatomy of upper abdominal organs, normal aortic locations, dimensions and content.

Test Outcome Deviations

- Presence of space-occupying lesions: cysts, solid masses, hematomas, abscesses, ascites, aneurysms, obstructions, arteriosclerotic changes to blood vessels.
- Organ size, location, or structural abnormalities.
- Biliary tract obstruction, dilation, calculi, hydronephrosis.

Interfering Factors

- Retained barium from prior radiographic studies will cause suboptimal results.

- Overlying intestinal gas will obscure organ visualization.
- Obesity adversely affects image quality.

Procedure

- A coupling medium, generally gel, is applied to the exposed abdomen in order to promote the transmission of sound. A hand-held transducer is slowly moved across the skin during this imaging procedure.
- The patient is instructed to control breathing pattern while the imaging is performed. Exam time is 30–60 minutes.
- Scans are performed in a variety of positions. Organ-specific sonograms (pancreas) can be performed.

Nursing Role

Use nursing process model following pre-, intra-, and posttest care guidelines in Chapter One. See page 8 for list of appropriate nursing diagnoses.

Nursing Diagnosis

- Knowledge deficit related to lack of information or possible misinterpretation of information provided about procedure.
- Anxiety and fear related to perception of diagnostic procedure as frightening or embarrassing.
- Powerlessness related to unfamiliar procedure, equipment.
- Ineffective coping related to test outcome and potential for surgery or other interventional techniques.

Pretest Care

- Explain exam purpose and procedure. Assure patient that no radiation is employed and that test is painless.
- Emphasize pretest food and drink restrictions. Patient should not consume any food 6–12 hours prior to test. Water is usually permitted.
- Administer enemas if ordered.
- Explain that a coupling gel will be applied to the skin. Although the couplant does not stain, advise patient to avoid wearing nonwashable clothing.

Intratest Care

- Encourage patient to follow breathing and positional instructions.

Posttest Care

- Remove or instruct patient to remove any residual gel from skin.
- Evaluate patient outcomes, provide support and counseling.

··············
CLINICAL ALERT

◊ Scans cannot be effectively performed over open wounds or dressings.
◊ This exam must be performed before or more than 24 hours after barium administration.
◊ Nonfasting will result in inadequate visualization of the gall bladder.
◊ Patient must agree to and sign a witnessed consent form prior to performance of an ultrasound-guided biopsy or other interventional procedures.
··············

ABO Red Cell Group

See Blood Groups and Types

Acid Phosphatase—Prostatic Acid Phosphatase (PAP)

See Tumor Markers

Adrenal Function Tests   Blood

These tests measure adrenal hormone function, insufficiency, and hyperfunction. Included are cortisol (hydrocortisone), cortisol suppression (dexamethasone suppression) (DST), and cortisol stimulation/cortrosyn stimulation.

Indications

- Evaluate Addison's disease and Cushing's syndrome.
- DST identifies persons most likely to respond to therapy.

Expected Test Outcomes

Cortisol

8:00 AM: 5–23 µg/dL or 1.38–6.35 µmol/L.
4:00 PM: 3–15 µg/dL or 83–414 µmol/L.

Cortisol suppression (DST)

8:00 AM: 6–26 µg/dL   morning after dexamethasone
4:00 PM: 2–18 µg/dL   administered: <5 µg/dL

Cortisol stimulation

Rise: >7 ng/dL   Peak: >20 ng/dL

Test Outcome Deviations

- *Cortisol increases* in oat-cell cancer, hyperthyroidism, adrenal adenoma, Cushing's disease.
- *Cortisol decreases* in liver disease, Addison's, anterior pituitary hyposecretion and destruction, hypothyroidism, and steroid therapy.

Interfering Factors for Cortisol

- Elevations in pregnancy, newborns, and some drugs (spironolactive and oral contraceptives).
- No diurnal variations in persons under stress.
- No *cortisol suppression* (DST) or diurnal variation in Cushing's and depressed persons.

Interfering Factors for Cortisol Suppression

- False positive if patient fails to take dexamethasone, drugs (dilantin, estrogen), anorexia, stress, trauma, dehydration, fever, and newborns.
- *No cortisol stimulation or blunted response* in adrenal insufficiency, hypopituitarism, and prolonged steroid therapy.

Procedure

- *Cortisol*: Serum (5 mL) samples obtained in the morning and evening. Collect by venipuncture, according to specimen collection guidelines in Chapter 2.
- *Cortisol suppression (DST)*: Serum samples obtained by venipuncture the day after oral administration of dexamethasone, later in the day. Dosage varies according to weight.
- *Cortisol stimulation*: Fasting serum (4 mL/obtained by venipuncture following specimen collection guidelines in Chapter 2). Give cortrosyn IM. Then collect additional 4-mL specimen 30 and 60 minutes after IM administration of cortrosyn.

Nursing Role

Use nursing process model following pre-, intra-, and posttest care guidelines in Chapter 1. See page 8 for list of appropriate nursing diagnoses.

Nursing Diagnosis

- Knowledge deficit related to lack or misinterpretation of information provided about purpose and procedure.
- High risk of injury (hematoma) or infection related to venipuncture and IM injection of cortrosyn.

Pretest Care

- Record accurate weight.
- Explain purpose and procedure. Remind about fasting for stimulant test.
- Check with physician and discontinue meds for 24–47 hours before study; especially aldosterone, estrogens, birth control meds, cortisone, tetracycline, and anticonvulsants.

Posttest Care

- Evaluate patient outcomes and counsel appropriately.

Alanine Aminotransferase (ALT); Serum Glutamic-Pyruvic Transaminase (SGPT)

See Liver Function Tests

Albumin

See Protein

Alcohol Ethanol (Ethyl), ETOH   Blood

This test detects and measures the presence of alcohol, as an indication of overdose and alcohol-impaired driving.

Indications

- Screen for alcohol in unconscious person.
- Assess levels for alcohol influence and alcohol intoxication.

Expected Test Outcomes

- Alcohol: None detected, negative.

Test Outcome Deviations

- At levels of 50–100 mg/dL, certain signs and symptoms are reported: flushing, slowing of reflexes, and impaired visual acuity. At levels higher than 100 mg/dL, central nervous system depression is reported. At levels >400 mg/dL, usually fatal.

Interfering Factors

- Increased blood ketones, as in diabetic ketoacidosis, can falsely elevate blood or breath test results.

···············
CLINICAL ALERT

◊ A value of greater than 300 mg/dL is a critical or panic value. Report and initiate overdose treatment at once.
◊ Proper collection, handling, and storage of the blood alcohol specimen is essential when the question of sobriety is raised. For legal purposes, "chain-of-custody" might have to be followed. See Chapter 2 regarding urine "chain-of-custody."
···············

Procedure

- Serum or plasma (5–7 mL) is obtained by venipuncture from arm in living persons. From dead persons, take samples from the aorta. DO NOT USE ALCOHOL TO CLEANSE THE AREA.
- A 20-mL sample of urine or gastric contents can be used.
- Breath analyzer measures ethanol content at end of expiration, following a deep inspiration.

Nursing Role

Use nursing process model following pre-, intra-, and posttest care guidelines in Chapter 1. See page 8 for list of appropriate nursing diagnoses.

Nursing Diagnosis

- Knowledge deficit related to lack or misinterpretation of information provided about purpose, procedure, and legal implications of testing for alcohol impaired driving.
- High risk for injury or infection related to venipuncture.

Pretest Care

- Explain purpose and procedure of test as proof of alcohol

influenced driving or intoxication. Check to see if informed consent must be signed prior to obtaining specimen.

Posttest Care

• Evaluate patient outcomes and monitor and counsel appropriately.

Aldolase

See Pancreatic Function Tests

Alkaline Phosphatase (ALP)

See Liver Function Tests

Allergens—IgE Antibodies

See RAST

Alpha-Fetoprotein (AFP)

See Amniotic Fluid Analysis and Tumor Markers

Alpha₁-Antitrypsin (AAT)   Blood

This test measures alpha₁-antitrypsin (protein produced by the liver), a deficiency of which is associated with pulmonary emphysema and other metabolic disorders.

Indications

• Evaluate respiratory disease and cirrhosis of liver.
• Screen for genetic deficiency with family history of emphysema.

Expected Test Outcomes

Alpha₁-antitrypsin level: 126–226 mg/dL

Test Outcome Deviations

• *Elevated levels* with inflammatory and hematological disorders and cancer.
• *Decreased levels* indicate early onset chronic pulmonary

emphysema in adults and liver cirrhosis in children; also severe liver damage and nephrotic syndrome.

Interfering Factors

- Pregnancy, stress, exercise, malnutrition, and oral contraceptives.
- Injections of typhoid vaccine will affect levels.

Procedure

- Serum (5 mL) obtained by venipuncture according to specimen collection guidelines in Chapter 2.
- Fasting is required if patient has elevated cholesterol or triglyceride levels.

Nursing Role

Use nursing process model following pre-, intra-, and posttest care guidelines in Chapter One. See page 8 for list of appropriate nursing diagnoses.

Nursing Diagnosis

- Knowledge deficit related to lack of information or possible misinterpretation of information provided about procedure, purpose and significance of decreased test outcomes and need for repeat testing.
- High risk for injury and/or infection related to venipuncture.

Pretest Care

- Explain purpose of test and instruct patient about fasting, if necessary.

Posttest Care

- Evaluate test outcomes and provide appropriate counseling.
- Explain to patient that further testing may be necessary if this protein is decreased. It involves pheno-typing the serum to assess significant risk of related disease such as pulmonary emphysema, liver cirrhosis.

Ammonia

See Liver Function Tests

Amniotic Fluid Analysis   Amniotic Fluid

Color, Volume, α-Fetoprotein (AFP), Creatinine, Lecithin
Sphingomyelin (LS) Ratio, Bilirubin

Amniotic fluid is examined *early* in pregnancy to study genetic makeup of the fetus and determine development abnormalities. Testing in third trimester is done to determine fetal age and well-being, study blood groups, and detect amnionitis.

Indications

- Offer prenatal diagnosis to high-risk parents to detect abnormal fetus.
- Evaluate hematologic disease, fetal infections, inborn metabolic disorders.
- Diagnose sex-linked disorders, chromosomal abnormalities and neural tube defects.

Expected Test Outcomes

Clear; fluid volumes of 30–1000 mL depending on stage of gestation.

AFP: age dependent; peak at 13–15 weeks = 30–43 µg/nL.

Creatinine: 1.5–2 mg/dL = fetal maturity.

L/S ratio: 2:1 or greater = pulmonary maturity.

        1:2 dilution (shake test) = lung maturity.

Bilirubin optical density: 0.02 or less indicates maturity.

Test Outcome Deviations

- Abnormal colors are associated with fetal distress, death, missed abortion, chromosomally abnormal fetus, anencephaly, and blood incompatibility.
- Increased volume in polyhydramnios are often associated with congenital abnormalities as esophageal atresia, anencephally, Rh disorder, and diabetes.
- Decreased volume in abnormal kidney function, premature rupture of membranes, intrauterine growth retardation.
- Creatinine decreases in prematurity.
- Increased bilirubin in impending fetal death.
- Elevated AFP indicates possible neural tube defects.
- Decreased AFP indicates fetal trisomy 21.
- Sickle cell anemia and thalassemia detected by fibroblast DNA examination.
- LS ratios decreased in pulmonary immaturity and respiratory distress syndrome.

Procedure

◇ Obtain a properly signed and witnessed consent form.

- Fetal position, viability, and number is assessed by ultrasound prior to amniotic tap. The tap site is away from the fetus, umbilical cord insertion, and any thick segment of placenta.
- A special needle is inserted through the abdominal wall into the amniotic sac. A 20–25 mL specimen is obtained and dressing is applied to needle site.

Nursing Role

Use nursing process model following pre-, intra-, and posttest care guidelines in Chapter One. See page 8 for list of appropriate nursing diagnoses.

Nursing Diagnosis

- Knowledge deficit related to lack of or misinterpretation of purpose and procedure.
- High risk of injury to fetus and infection related to amniocentesis.
- Ineffective coping (individual and/or family) related to test outcome.

Pretest Care

- Explain purpose and risks of prenatal diagnosis procedure, and assess for contraindications: premature labor history, incompetent cervix, placenta previa, or abruptio placenta.
- Obtain baseline BP, pulse, respiration, and fetal heart rate.

Intratest Care

- Provide support and reassurance during the procedure.
- Nausea, vertigo, and mild cramps may occur.

Posttest Care

- Evaluate patient outcomes and counsel appropriately in collaboration with physician. Results are not infallible and outcomes may not reflect true fetal status.
- Monitor for complications: spontaneous abortion, fetal injury, hemorrhage, infection, and Rh sensitivity if fetal blood enters mother's circulation.

Amylase Excretion, Clearance

See Pancreatic Function Tests

Antibody to Human Immunodeficiency Virus (HIV); Acquired Immunodeficiency Syndrome (AIDS) Test

Blood

This test is done to diagnose acquired immunodeficiency syndrome (AIDS), a clinical syndrome which develops following infection by human immunodeficiency virus (HIV).

Indications

- Evaluate suspected infection with HIV and assess patients with history of high-risk exposure to HIV-infected persons, either through sexual or parenteral activities.
- Screen persons whose blood and plasma products are being donated for transfusion.

Procedure

- Serum (5 mL) obtained by venipuncture according to specimen collection guidelines in Chapter 2.

Expected Test Outcomes

Negative: Nonreactive for antibody to HIV.

Test Outcome Deviations

- A positive test should be repeated and confirmed by other tests.
- An ELISA test is used as a screening procedure and, if positive, must be followed by a Western Blot to confirm the presence of antibody to HIV.
- A positive result may occur in noninfected persons due to unknown factors.
- A negative test tends to rule out AIDS as a diagnosis for high-risk patients with illness but who do not have characteristic opportunistic infection or tumor.

Interfering Factors

- Nonreactive HIV test results occur during acute stage of infection when virus is present but antibody development is

not sufficient to be detected. Virus may be present for up to 6 months before antibody can be detected. During this stage the test for HIV antigen may confirm an HIV infection.
- Nonspecific reactions may occur with prior pregnancy or blood transfusions.

Nursing Role

Use nursing process model following pre-, intra-, and posttest care guidelines in Chapter 1. See page 8 for list of appropriate nursing diagnoses.

Nursing Diagnosis

- Knowledge deficit related to purpose, procedure, and confidentiality of test results.
- High risk of infection or injury, bleeding or hematoma related to venipuncture.
- Anxiety and fear related to test outcome and possible diagnosis of AIDS.

Pretest Care

- Assess patient's knowledge of test and test procedure.

••••••••••••••
CLINICAL ALERT

◊ An informed consent must be signed by any person who is being tested for AIDS. The consent must accompany specimen to the laboratory or, if patient goes to the laboratory for venipuncture, consent must accompany patient.
◊ It is essential that counseling precede and follow administration of an HIV antibody test. Test should not be performed without the subject's prior knowledge. The informed-consent process should include a discussion of clinical and behavioral implications of test results, including accuracy of the test and encouragement of behavioral changes (eg, sexual contact, shared needles, or blood transfusion). The person tested must also be aware of other people to whom test results must be given, such as those health care workers who have legitimate access to patient charts.
◊ The physician must sign a legal form stating that patient has been informed of the risks of testing.
••••••••••••••

Posttest Care

- Evaluate patient outcomes and counsel appropriately.

- Results should not be given by telephone. Use of computer for transmission of results varies in medical facilities. Check with your facility for current regulation regarding use of computer for HIV test results.
- All results, both positive and negative, must be documented in health care record. Precautions must be taken to maintain confidentiality of results. People are more likely to undergo testing voluntarily if they believe that inappropriate disclosure of HIV testing information, which could result in loss of job, housing, or insurance coverage, will not occur.
- Recognizing HIV infection as a disease is important. Drugs are being tested to determine whether they halt or slow the disease process in infected asymptomatic individuals. Treatments for infections and malignancies that occur in AIDS patients are more effective and less toxic when started early in the course of HIV infection.
- A person who has antibodies to HIV is presumed infected with the virus, and appropriate counseling and medical evaluation should be offered.
- Positive test results must be reported to the state public health authorities following regulations established in each state.

Antinuclear Antibodies   Blood

Antinuclear Antibody (ANA), Antideoxyribonucleic Acid (DNA) Antibody (Anti-DNA), Anti-ds-Double Stranded DNA Antibody

These tests measure and differentiate antinuclear antibodies associated with certain autoimmune diseases, especially systemic lupus erythematosus (SLE) and related connective tissue disease.

Indications

- Diagnose SLE.
- Differentiate SLE from rheumatoid arthritis and other systemic autoimmune disorders.
- Monitor therapy and establish treatment program for SLE.

Expected Test Outcomes

ANA Titer: Negative; Anti-ds-DNA: < 70 units (ELISA); < 1:20 (IFA); < 12% bound (FARR); Anti-DNA antibodies: 70 units (ELISA); 1:20 (IFA); < 12% bound (FARR).

Test Outcome Deviations

- ANA positive at a titer of 1:20 or 1:40, depending on the laboratory. The higher the titer, the more specific to diagnosing SLE.
- A positive result does not necessarily indicate a disease process because ANAs are present in some apparently healthy persons. Some positive reactions have been reported to be related to patients with connective tissue disease (SLE, lupoid hepatitis, scleroderma, rheumatoid arthritis, and discoid lupus, Sjögren's dermatomyositis, and polyarteritis) or to persons who may develop such a disease at a later time.
- A negative test for total ANA is strong evidence against the diagnosis of SLE.
- Anti-DNA and anti-ds-DNA increased in acute recurrence of SLE (anti-DNA immune complexes play an active role in pathogenesis of SLE through the deposit of the complexes in the kidney and other tissues), and may indicate presence of other autoimmune diseases.
- Decrease in elevated anti-DNA and anti-ds-DNA following immunosuppressive therapy may indicate effective treatment of SLE.

Interfering Factors

- A radioactive scan performed within 1 week of collecting blood sample may alter anti-DNA test results.
- Age, smoking, and a number of drugs cause positive test for ANAs. Patients receiving anticonvulsants, oral contraceptives, and procainamide or hydralazine, for example, may develop ANAs at increased titers even though they may not exhibit any clinical features of SLE.

Procedure

- Serum (5–10 mL) obtained by venipuncture according to specimen collection guidelines in Chapter 2.
- List patient's drugs that can affect test results on laboratory slip or computer screen.

Nursing Role

Use nursing process model following pre-, intra-, and posttest care guidelines in Chapter One. See page 8 for list of appropriate nursing diagnoses.

Nursing Diagnosis

- Knowledge deficit related to lack or possible misinterpretation of information provided about procedure and purpose.
- High risk for injury/infection related to venipuncture.
- Knowledge deficit related to test outcome deviation that may necessitate medication or life-style alterations.

Pretest Care

- Assess patient's knowledge of test and cardiac medication usage such as procainamide and hydralazine which cause SLE-like symptoms.
- Explain purpose of blood test is to determine presence of connective-tissue disorder—no fasting is required.

Posttest Care

- Evaluate patient outcomes, monitor and counsel appropriately. Prepare for possibility of repeat testing (anti-ds-DNA increases or decreases according to disease activity and response to therapy).
- Observe venipuncture site for signs of infection (patients with autoimmune disease have a compromised immune system).
- Advise patient that minor symptoms of SLE (without major organ involvement) are treated with nonsteroidal anti-inflammatory drugs such as salicylates. Short-acting corticosteroids, such as prednisone, are necessary if acute serologic changes (e.g., increased ANA titer) and severe clinical manifestations occur. Side effects are minimal. Long-term, moderate-to-high dose corticosteroid therapy is required for diffuse proliferative glomerulonephritis. Side effects are more pronounced.

Arterial Blood Gases (ABGs)   Blood
Blood Gases

pH, $PaCO_2$, HCO_3, SaO_2, and PaO_2

Arterial blood is analyzed to assess adequacy of oxygenation, ventilation, and acid-base status.

Indications

- Evaluate ventilatory and acid-base disturbances and monitor effectiveness of therapy.

- Titrate the appropriate oxygen flow rate.
- Qualify a patient for home-oxygen use.

Expected Test Outcomes

- pH = negative log of the hydrogen ion concentration: Adult: 7.35–7.45; child: 7.36–7.44.
- $PaCO_2$ = partial pressure of carbon dioxide: 35–45 mm Hg or torr.
- HCO_3 = bicarbonate concentration: 22–28 mEq/L.
- SaO_2 = percent of hemoglobin carrying oxygen: > 95%, oxygen saturation.
- PaO_2 = partial pressure of oxygen: >80 mm Hg or torr.

Test Outcome Deviations

Blood gas values outside of the above ranges can be grouped into two primary and four underlying disturbances for interpretive basis.

VENTILATORY DISTURBANCE	pH	$PaCO_2$	HCO_3
1. Respiratory acidosis	Decrease	Increase	Normal
Compensated	Normal	Increase	Increase
2. Respiratory alkalosis	Increase	Decrease	Normal
Compensated	Normal	Decrease	Decrease
ACID-BASE DISTURBANCE			
3. Metabolic acidosis	Decrease	Normal	Decrease
Compensated	Normal	Decrease	Decrease
4. Metabolic alkalosis	Increase	Normal	Increase
Compensated	Normal	Increase	Increase

· · · · · · · · · · · · ·
CLINICAL ALERT

◇ Although there are four basic disturbances, a combined disturbance is generally the case. More recent terminology refers to the uncompensated disturbances as "acute" and the compensated as "chronic." Also, the term metabolic has been replaced with the term "nonrespiratory." Decreases in the PaO_2 are interpreted separately and referred to as hypoxemia.
· · · · · · · · · · · · ·

Interfering Factors

- Recent smoking can increase the carboxyhemoglobin level, thereby decreasing the SaO_2 with little to no effect on the PaO_2.

- Although supplemental oxygen will increase the PaO_2, it can also cause CO_2 retention due to a decrease in ventilatory drive via the hypoxic stimulus.

Procedure

- Arterial blood specimen of 3–5 mL is obtained in a heparinized syringe. See specimen collection guidelines in Chapter 2.
- Label tube or syringe with patient's name, identification number, date, time, whether on room air or oxygen and rate of flow.
- The results are reported (some laboratories analyze the sample twice and report the average) and compared against established laboratory or clinical ranges.

••••••••••••••
CLINICAL ALERT

◊ Call the laboratory if sample cannot be analyzed within 10 minutes; place in ice. An iced blood gas sample should be analyzed within 1 hour. Longer delays can result in changes in oxygen, carbon dioxide, and pH levels.
••••••••••••••

Nursing Role

Use nursing process model following pre-, intra-, and posttest care guidelines in Chapter 1. See page 8 for list of appropriate nursing diagnoses.

Nursing Diagnosis

- Knowledge deficit related to lack of information or misinterpretation of information provided about purpose and procedure of ABGs.
- Fear or anxiety related to arterial puncture.
- High risk of injury, bleeding, or infection related to arterial puncture.
- Discomfort or pain related to arterial puncture.

Pretest Care

- Explain purpose and procedure of ABG. As this is an invasive procedure, the patient may express concern and be somewhat apprehensive.
- Assure patient that arterial puncture is similar to other blood tests she/he may have had and that a local anesthetic can be used if desired. If near mealtime, encourage the patient to eat.

Intratest Care

- The arterial puncture can cause some discomfort and if patient is nervous or apprehensive, a local anesthetic (1% lidocaine) can be used. Prior to injection, assess for allergy to the anesthetic.
- During procedure, if patient experiences a dull or sharp pain radiating up the arm, the needle should be withdrawn slightly and repositioned. If repositioning does not alleviate pain, the needle should be completely withdrawn.
- Be aware that some patients may experience light-headedness, nausea, and in some cases vasovagal syncope, and be ready to respond appropriately.

Posttest Care

- Observe frequently for bleeding. A pressure dressing should be applied if necessary. Apply pressure to the site for a couple of minutes.
- Evaluate patient outcomes; assess and monitor appropriately for hypoxemia, ventilatory, and acid-base disturbances.

●●●●●●●●●●●●●●
CLINICAL ALERT
◊ See Appendix C for standards of critical (panic) values.
●●●●●●●●●●●●●●

Arthrogram
Arthrography
X-Ray Imaging with Contrast

An arthrogram is an x-ray procedure that can be used to demonstrate the soft tissue structures of joints. Knee, ankle, shoulder, hip and wrist arthrograms are commonly performed.

Indications

- Evaluation of persistent unexplained joint pain.
- Evaluate cartilage, tendons, ligaments.

Procedure

- A local anesthetic is injected in the surrounding tissues. A needle is placed into the joint space. Fluid from the joint may be aspirated. An iodinated contrast agent is introduced into the joint space. Following needle removal, the joint is manipulated to distribute the contrast material. X-ray films are taken of the joint in several positions.

- Procedure time is generally less than 1 hour.

Expected Test Outcomes

Normal joint space, bursae, ligaments, cartilage and tendons.

Test Outcome Deviations

- Narrowing of joint space, dislocation, tear or rupture of ligaments, cartilage, tendons, and cysts.

Interfering Factors

- Metallic objects which overlie the area of interest will interfere with organ visualization.
- Severe obesity adversely affects image quality.

Nursing Role

Use nursing process model following pre-, intra-, and posttest care guidelines in Chapter 1. See page 8 for list of appropriate nursing diagnoses.

Nursing Diagnosis

- Knowledge deficit related to lack of information or possible misinterpretation of information provided about the procedure or purpose.
- Anxiety and fear related to unfamiliarity with diagnostic procedure and equipment.
- High risk for injury related to administration of contrast medium.
- Pain related to arthrogram procedure.

Pretest Care

- Assess for test contraindications: pregnancy, sensitivity to iodine. Explain exam purpose and procedure, and make certain that jewelry and metallic objects are removed from the joint to be examined. See Appendix A for standards for contrast media precautions.

••••••••••••••
CLINICAL ALERT

◊ Obtain a signed informed consent form.
••••••••••••••

Intratest Care

- Provide support during needle placement. Some discomfort is to be expected.

- Encourage patient to follow positional instructions during contrast manipulation and x-ray exposures.

Posttest Care
- Evaluate patient outcome and monitor appropriately.
- An elastic bandage may be applied to knee joint for several days; ice packs or analgesics may be used to alleviate pain.
- Check for complications at injection site.
- Cracking or clicking noises may be heard in the joint for several days.

Arthroscopy   Endoscopic Imaging

Arthroscopy is a visual examination of a joint with a fiberoptic endoscope.

Indications
- Detect and diagnose diseases and injuries of the meniscus, patella, condyle, extrasynovial area, and synovium.
- Assess degenerative processes and response to treatments.
- Perform arthroscopic surgery.

Expected Test Outcomes

Normal joints, vasculature, and synovium capsule, menisci, tendons, ligaments, and articular cartilage.

Test Outcome Deviations
- Torn or displaced meniscus or cartilage, trapped synovium, loose fragments of joint components, torn or ruptured ligaments, nerve entrapment, fractures, non-union of fractures, and subluxation.
- Degenerative disease, osteochondritis, osteoarthritis, inflammatory arthritis, osteochondritis dissecans (cartilage and bone detach from the articular surface), chondromalacia, cysts, ganglions, and infections.

Interfering Factors
- Presence of ankylosis, fibrosis, sepsis, or contrast medium in joint from previous arthrogram.

Procedure
- Under general, local, or spinal anesthesia, an arthroscope is inserted into the joint through a small incision after a tourni-

quet is applied to the area. After the joint is aspirated, a continuous irrigation flushes the joint during the procedure. Specimens are retrieved from the flush solution.

- Photographs and videotapes are frequently obtained during the process. The joint is compressed as instruments are withdrawn, to expel irrigant. Steroids or local anesthetics may be injected into the joint at end of the case. The wound is closed and dressed; splints or immobilizers may be applied.

Nursing Role

Use nursing process model following pre-, intra-, and posttest care guidelines in Chapter 1. See page 8 for list of appropriate nursing diagnoses.

Nursing Diagnosis

- Potential for altered tissue perfusion related to edema or constrictive dressing.
- Pain related to effects of arthroscopic procedure.
- Impaired physical mobility related to perception of pain upon movement.

Pretest Care

- Explain the purpose and procedure. Patient should fast from midnight before procedure, unless otherwise ordered.

••••••••••••
CLINICAL ALERT
◇ Obtain a properly signed and witnessed consent form.
••••••••••••

- Requisite lab work, x-rays, history and physical exam, and other test results should be charted. Inform physician of abnormal results.
- Check pulses on the operative extremity. Take baseline vital signs.
- Teach crutch-walking and other postprocedure regimens.

Intratest Care

- Follow usual protocols for arthroscopic procedures in operative environment.

Posttest Care

- Recover patient according to protocols. Include frequent vital signs and wound checks. Do neurovascular checks of affected extremity (color, temperature, motion, sensation, pulses, and capillary refill times).

- Administer pain medication as needed/ordered and ice and elevation to the affected area if ordered.
- Frequently, these cases are scheduled as ambulatory surgery; follow protocols for discharge. Instruct patient to report numbness, tingling, coldness, duskiness, swelling, bleeding, or abnormally severe pain to physician STAT. Mild soreness and mild grinding sensation for a few days is normal. However, signs of infection and fever should be reported to the physician promptly.

. . . .
CLINICAL ALERTS

◊ In elevating the leg, make sure *entire* leg is elevated in a straight position. If knee is flexed, a flexion contracture may result.

◊ Signs of thrombophlebitis include calf tenderness, pain, and warmth. Instruct patient to report these symptoms STAT. **Do Not Massage the Area**.

◊ Compartment syndrome is a musculoskeletal complication that occurs most frequently in the forearm or leg. Fascia surrounding the muscle does not expand in the presence of edema or swelling, and the neurovascular status of the extremity is compromised. This is an emergency situation and usually requires surgical intervention to release pressure.

. . . .

Aspartate Aminotransferase (AST)

See Cardiac Enzymes

Barium Enema— (Large Bowel Study, Colon X-Ray)

Air Contrast Enema
X-Ray Imaging with Contrast

This exam uses both x-ray and fluoroscopic techniques to demonstrate the anatomy of the large intestine.

Indications

- Rule out obstruction, polyps, diverticula or other masses, fistula, and inflammatory changes.
- Evaluate bowel change and abdominal pain.

Expected Test Outcomes

Normal position, contour, filling, and patency of the large bowel.

Test Outcome Deviations

- Congenital deformities, bowel obstruction, stenosis, lesions such as diverticula, polyps, tumors, fistulas, hernia, inflammatory changes such as colitis, and appendicitis.

Procedure

- Patient is given a contrast agent (usually barium) in the form of an enema via the rectum or through an ostomy. Under fluoroscopy, colon is completely filled to the ileo-cecal junction. For a satisfactory examination, the contrast-filled colon must be maintained for several minutes while x-rays are taken. In some instances, air is also introduced into the colon (the so-called air contrast or double contrast enema).
- Patient is instructed to retain barium while films are taken with patient in a variety of positions. After filming is completed, patient is asked to go into the bathroom and expel the barium. A post-evacuation film is then taken to document colon emptying. Total exam time is approximately 30–60 minutes.

Interfering Factors

- Retained fecal material caused by poor/inadequate bowel cleansing.
- Inability of patient to maintain contrast-filled colon long enough to allow complete examination.
- Severe obesity adversely affects image quality.

Nursing Role

Use nursing process model following pre-, intra-, and posttest care guidelines in Chapter 1. See page 8 for list of appropriate nursing diagnoses.

Nursing Diagnosis

- Knowledge deficit related to lack or possible misinterpretation of information provided about procedure or purpose.
- Anxiety and fear related to unfamiliarity with diagnostic procedure and equipment.
- Ineffective coping related to test outcome and inability to accept diagnosis of bowel disease.

- High risk of injury related to reaction to barium contrast.

Pretest Care

- Assess for test contraindications (pregnancy). Explain exam purpose and procedure. Assure patient that amount of time needed to maintain a full colon is relatively short (generally just a few minutes).
- No food or beverage is allowed for approximately 8 hours prior to study. Make certain that jewelry and metallic objects are removed from abdominal area.
- Bowel preparation routines will vary and may involve any combination of clear liquid diet preceding test, cleansing enemas, and stool softeners/laxatives.
- See Appendix A for standards regarding contrast media precautions.

Intratest Care

- Encourage patient to follow breathing and positional instructions.

Posttest Care

- Provide fluids, food, and rest after study. Administer laxatives if ordered.
- Observe and record stool color/consistency to determine if all barium has been eliminated from the bowel.
- Evaluate patient outcomes; provide support and counseling.

··············
CLINICAL ALERT

◊ The use of barium is contraindicated when bowel perforation is suspected. A water-soluble, iodinated contrast is substituted for barium in this instance.
◊ Use of cathartics or enemas may be contraindicated with ulcerative colitis or obstruction. Patients with toxic megacolon should not be given enemas. Special consideration must be made for patients with ostomies. Consult physician or radiology department in case of questions regarding bowel preparation.
··············

Basophils

See Complete Blood Count (CBC)

Bicarbonate

See Arterial Blood Gases (ABGs)

Bilirubin

See Liver Function Tests

Blastomycosis

See Fungal Antibody Tests

Bleeding Time

See Coagulation Studies

Blood Culture   Blood

A blood culture is done to identify the specific microorganism that is causing a clinical infection.

Indications
- Evaluate bacteremia and septicemia and effectiveness of antibiotic therapy.
- Investigate unexplained postoperative shock and chills and fever of more than several days duration.

Expected Test Outcomes
Negative cultures for aerobic or anaerobic organisms.

Test Outcome Deviations
- Positive cultures and identification of pathogens most common are: *Staphylococcus aureus, Escherichia coli, Enterococcus (Streptoccus D), Streptoccus pneumoniae, Klebsiella pneumoniae, Klebsiella pneumoniae, Streptoccus pyogenes (Streptoccus A)* and *Pseudomonas, Candida albicans and Anaerobic fragilis.*
- True infection is almost always present if organism is streptococcus of the nonveridans group.

Interfering Factors
- Contamination of specimen due to skin bacteria; nonfilter-

able blood usually due to presence of abnormal proteins and
antibacterial therapy affect.

Procedure

- Blood (20–30 mL) obtained by venipuncture according to
  specimen collection guidelines in Chapter 2. Collect 2–3 cultures at least 30–60 minutes apart (if possible) per 24-hour
  period. Obtain as soon as possible after onset of chills and
  fever and before starting antibiotic therapy. Do not draw
  blood from IV catheter unless no vein sites are available.
- Observe rigorous aseptic technique as the potential for infect-
  ing patient as a result of venipuncture is very high. Scrub
  puncture site with Betadine (providine-iodine); allow to dry;
  then cleanse with 70% alcohol.
- On laboratory slip or on computer screen, note patient's age;
  this alerts laboratory to age-related pathogens.
- Note diagnosis because immunosuppressed patients are
  infected by organisms that rarely invade the healthy person.
- Note if IV line has been present longer than 48 hours which
  helps to correctly assess significance of uncommon pathogens.

Nursing Role

Use nursing process model following pre-, intra-, and posttest
care guidelines in Chapter 1. See page 8 for list of appropriate
nursing diagnoses.

Nursing Diagnosis

- Knowledge deficit related to lack of information or possible
  misinterpretation of information provided about the procedure and purpose.
- High risk for injury and/or infection related to venipuncture.
- Knowledge deficit related to significance of positive culture
  and required medical/nursing intervention necessary to treat
  infection or prevent further transmission of disease to others.

Pretest Care

- Assess patient's knowledge of test and medication use
  (specifically, antibiotics). Explain purpose and timing of
  blood test procedure. No fasting is required.

Intratest Care

- Cleanse top(s) of culture bottle(s) with iodine and allow to
  dry before putting in specimen. Bottle or vacuum tubes

should contain a culture medium. If two bottles are used (anaerobic and aerobic), inoculate anaerobic first with enough blood to have 1:10 dilution in blood: broth mixture. Then inoculate aerobic bottle with the same dilution.

Posttest Care

- Send specimen to lab immediately. Label with patient's name, age, date, time, number of culture, notation of patient isolation category, and if on antibiotics.
- Counsel patient regarding positive results and possible need for further testing to identify where infection is located in the body, to further validate results, or to evaluate effectiveness of therapy.

••••••••••••••
CLINICAL ALERT

◊ Counsel patient regarding the significance of completing medical regimen (antibiotic therapy).
◊ Notify physician at once of positive culture.
••••••••••••••

Blood Glucose/Sugar Tests   **Blood**

*Fasting Blood Sugar (FBS), 2-h Post-Prandial Blood Sugar (PPBS),
Oral Glucose Tolerance Test (OGTT, GTT),
Glycosylated Hemoglobin*

These tests measure glucose concentration, carbohydrate metabolism, glucose tolerance, instability, control, and aid in diabetes management.

Indications

- Screen for and rule out diabetes and hypoglycemia.
- Diagnose borderline abnormalities of glucose tolerance.
- Index of long-term glucose control (glycosylated hemoglobin).

Expected Test Outcomes

FBS:	FASTING	GLYCOSYLATED HEMOGLOBIN
Adult	70–110 mg/dL serum or plasma	Nondiabetic: 4.0%–7.0%
Elderly	70–120 mg/dL serum	Diabetic: >7.0%

Child   60–100 mg/dL serum   Results expressed as % of
                                   total hemoglobin
Newborn   30–80 mg/dL serum

2-h PPBS: After a meal, less than 65–139 mg/dL/2 h
OGTT: FBS < 115 mg/dL or < 64 mmol/L
90 minutes: < 200 mg/dL or < 11.1 mmol/L
2 hours: < 140 mg/dL or 7.8 mmol/L

Test Outcome Deviations

- Abnormal values are indicative of type 1: insulin-dependent diabetes mellitus (IDDM); type 2: non–insulin-dependent diabetes mellitus (NIDDM); type 3: gestational diabetes; type 4: impaired glucose tolerance; type 5: potential abnormality of glucose tolerance; and type 6: glucose intolerance associated with certain conditions and syndromes.

Test Outcome Deviations: FBS

- World Health Organization defines hyperglycemia increases of fasting glucose as 140 mg/dL or greater in more than one occasion or any glucose of 200 mg/dL or greater. Hypoglycemia is defined as glucose less than 50 mg/dL in men and less than 40 mg/dL in women.
- *Increases (hyperglycemia)* in diabetes mellitus states of increased circulating epinephrine, acute pancreatitis, vitamin B_1 deficiency, subarachnoid hemorrhage, and convulsive states.
- *Decreases (hypoglycemia)* in pancreatic disorders as islet cell tumors, cancers of stomach and adrenal gland, liver disease, postgastrectomy and pediatric anomalies, and enzyme diseases, among others.

Interfering Factors, FBS

- Increases caused by many drugs, diuretics, cortisone, estrogen, anticonvulsants, pregnancy, stress, adrenal infections, and anesthesia.

Test Outcome Deviations: PPBS

- *Increases in PPBS* greater than 200 mg/dL is consistent with a diagnosis of diabetes mellitus.
- *Increases* in many stressful and serious conditions as malnutrition, advanced cirrhosis, Cushing's syndrome, hyperthyroidism, myocardial or cerebral infarction, and hypoproteinemias.

- *Decreases in PPBS* in anterior pituitary insufficiency, islet cell adenoma, steatorrhea, Addison's disease, and rapid stomach emptying.

Interfering Factors, PPBS

- Smoking and coffee cause increases.

Test Outcome Deviations: OGTT

- Diabetic glucose tolerance: Fasting: < 140 mg/dL; 2 h: > 200 mg/dL; $1/2$, 1, or $11/2$ h: > 200 mg/dL.
- Gestational diabetes (2 or more must be met and exceeded). Fasting > 105 mg/dL; 1 h: > 190 mg/dL; 2 h: > 165 mg/dL; 3 h: > 145 mg/dL.
- Impaired glucose tolerance (IGT) all 3 must be met. Fasting: < 140 mg/dL; 2 h: 140–200 mg/dL; $1/2$, 1 or $11/2$ h: > 200 mg/dL.
- Values above normals but below criteria for diabetes or IGT are not diagnostic for these conditions.
- *Increased tolerance* (excessive peak) in gastrectomy, hyperthyroidism, diabetes mellitus, hyperlipedemia, hemochromatosis, Cushing's disease, CNS lesions, and severe liver disease.
- *Decreased tolerance* (flat peak) in pancreatic islet cells, hyperplasia or tumor, intestinal diseases, hypothyroidism, and liver disease.

Interfering Factors, OGTT

- Smoking, weight reducing diets, prolonged bed rest, infectious diseases, and many drugs affect outcomes.

Test Outcome Deviations: Glycosylated Hemoglobin

- Good control < 7%; fair control 8–12%; poor control 13–20%.
- *Increases* in chronic renal failure, iron deficiency anemia, splenectomy, alcohol and lead toxicity.

Interfering Factors—Glycosylated Hemoglobin

- Decrease in pregnancy, hemolytic anemia, and chronic blood loss.

Procedures

FBS Procedure

- Sample is taken after overnight fast. Collect plasma (5–10 mL) by venipuncture, according to guidelines in Chapter 2.
- Note drugs patient is taking on lab slip or computer screen.

PPBS Procedure

- Blood sample taken after overnight fast and a high carbohydrate breakfast. Record time breakfast is completed and notify laboratory. Two hours after breakfast is finished, a venous sample (5 mL) is collected following guidelines in Chapter 2.
- Note drugs patient is taking on lab slip or computer screen.

OGGT Procedure

- Test done in morning after overnight fast: 2 hours for diabetes check in men and non-pregnant women; 3 hours for pregnancy; 1/2 hour for hypoglycemia. A fasting blood sample and urine are obtained. Patient drinks a commercial glucose liquid. Blood (5 mL) and urine specimens are obtained at intervals and collected according to guidelines in Chapter 2.
- Document drugs that affect outcomes. Check with physician about administering salicylates, diuretics, and hormones before test.

Glycosylated Hemoglobin Procedure

- A blood sample with EDTA anticoagulant (3 mL) is obtained by venipuncture, following specimen collection guidelines in Chapter 2.

Nursing Role

Use nursing process model following pre-, intra-, and posttest care guidelines in Chapter 1. See page 8 for list of appropriate nursing diagnoses.

Nursing Diagnosis

- Knowledge deficit related to lack or misinterpretation of information provided about purpose, procedure, and need for patient cooperation.
- High risk of injury, hematoma, bleeding, or infection related to venipuncture.
- Potential for noncompliance to test protocols related to inability to follow instructions.
- Ineffective individual coping related to test outcomes and inability to accept diagnosis of serious disease.

• • • • • • • • • • • • • •
CLINICAL ALERT

◊ Postpone GTT in unexpected illnesses with fever or GI upsets or if ingestion of food within 8 hours.

◊ If FBS is over 200, the glucose tolerance is usually not done. If it is, monitor patient for severe reaction or onset of coma.
◊ See Appendix C for standards of critical (panic) values.

•••••••••••••

Pretest Care

- Explain purposes, indications, procedures, and interfering factors of tests. All are fasting except post-prandial which is feasting (after eating). Assess for smoking, history of recent weight reduction, and current meds.
- Note that post-prandial timed test is contraindicated in obvious diabetes mellitus. Glucose tolerance limited test is contraindicated for patients on bed rest, and following recent surgery, myocardial infarction, and labor and delivery.

Intratest Care

- For timed tests, patients should be at rest, not walking about, and no eating or smoking; water only. If patient vomits glucose, test is invalid and has to be repeated after 3 days.
- Record reactions during GTT: weakness, faintness, sweating may occur during second and third hours. If this occurs, obtain blood sample immediately and discontinue test.

Posttest Care

- Patient may eat and drink as soon as test is over. Diabetics may have insulin and oral hypoglycemics when tests are completed.
- Evaluate patient outcomes, monitor, and counsel appropriately. Provide information, support, and comfort if diagnosis of diabetes mellitus.

Blood in Stool

See Stool Analysis

Blood Groups and Types   Blood

Crossmatch Compatibility, Rh Factors, Coombs,
ABO Groups, Antibody Titer and Screens

This series of tests is done to prevent transfusion of incompatible blood products and transplant reactions, to confirm ABO grouping by examining RBCs for presence of blood group antigens and RBCs and antibodies against these antigens.

Indications

- Required of blood donors and potential blood recipients.
- Determine parentage.
- Detect and prevent hemolytic newborn disease and Rh typing when woman has had abortion or miscarriage.
- Before surgery that may require transfusion, crossmatch to detect antibodies to *recipient's* serum that damage *donor* cells (major crossmatch), or detect antibodies in *donor's* cells that may affect RBCs of *recipient* (minor crossmatch).

Expected Test Outcomes

- Adult: *Compatibility*: Absence of agglutination (clumping) of cells.
  Rh: *White*: 85% Rh positive; 15% Rh negative.
  Black: 90% Rh positive; 10% Rh negative.
- Rh antibody titer: Normal is zero; no antibody.
- Coombs test: Direct and indirect: Negative.
- Blood group: A, B, AB, O.
- Child: Same as adult.
- Antibody screen: Negative (implies that recipient can receive type-specific ABO-Rh identical blood with minimal risk).

Test Outcome Deviations

- Incompatibility: presence of agglutination (clumping) of cells.
- Rh antibody titer: presence of unusual antibodies or titer in pregnant women greater than 1:64 (requires transfusion exchange).
- Coombs test: *direct-positive* (1+ to 4+) incompatible crossmatch blood, specific antibody (previous transfusion, anti-Rh antibodies, acquired hemolytic anemia). *Indirect-positive* (1+ to 4+) erythroblastosis fetalis, hemolytic anemia (autoimmune or drugs), transfusion hemolytic reactions (blood incompatibility, leukemia), systemic lupus erythematosus.

Procedure

- Collect clotted blood specimen (10 mL) for groups or types by venipuncture according to guidelines in chapter 2. Red cells are examined.
- For antibody screens and crossmatch, plasma or serum is the specimen.
- Include as appropriate the diagnosis, history of recent and past transfusions, pregnancy, and drug therapy.

Nursing Role

Use nursing process model following pre-, intra-, and posttest care guidelines in Chapter 1. See page 8 for list of appropriate nursing diagnoses.

Nursing Diagnosis

- Knowledge deficit related to lack of information or possible misinterpretation of information provided about procedure, equipment, purpose, and preparation.
- High risk for injury, bleeding, hematoma, or infection related to venipuncture.
- Potential decisional conflict related to test outcomes.
- Ineffective individual/family coping related to test outcome and acceptance of diagnosis of potential disease in newborn.

Pretest Care

- Explain purpose and procedure—no fasting is required.
- Explain the relation of test to potential serious transfusion reactions.
- Recognize need for follow-up testing in prenatal screening of Rh-antibody if titer is negative (repeat 30–36 weeks of pregnancy).
- List drugs patient is taking on lab slip or computer screen (especially for Coombs test).

Posttest Care

- Monitor venipuncture sites for signs of bleeding or infection—apply pressure dressing to site.
- If Coombs test is positive, antibody identification is then done.
- In addition to blood specimen, saliva, semen, and cervical mucus specimens may be tested to identify blood groupings (paternity issues).
- Evaluate patient's outcomes and counsel appropriately, including advising mother of the need for RhoGam to prevent further hemolytic problems.
- Assess for possible transfusion reaction, even when giving compatible blood.

• • • • • • • • • • • • •
CLINICAL ALERTS

◊ Required tests for all blood donors include: ABO red cell group, Rh factor, antibody screen, test for hepatitis B surface antigen (HB5 Ag), test for non-A non-B hepatitis, alanine aminotransferase (ALT) test for hepatitis C virus (anti-HVC), test for syphilis (VDRL), test for acquired immune deficiency syndrome (HIV), and test for adult T-cell leukemia/lymphoma (HTLV-I). [Cytomegalovirus (CMV) testing is done for immunosuppressive persons].

• • • • • • • • • • • • •

Blood pH

See Arterial Blood Gases

Blood Sugar

See Blood Glucose Tests
See Arterial Blood Gases (ABGs)

Blood Urea Nitrogen (BUN)

See Kidney Function Tests

Bone Marrow Aspiration or Biopsy

Bone Marrow

A bone marrow specimen is obtained through aspiration or needle biopsy to fully evaluate blood cell formation (hematopoiesis).

Indications

• Diagnose hemolytic blood disorders by analyzing cell number appearance, development, presence of infection, and deficiency states of vitamin B_{12}, folic acid, iron, and pyridoxine.
• Diagnose primary and metastatic tumors, infectious diseases, certain granulomas, and aid in diagnosis and staging process of malignancies.
• Isolate bacteria or other pathogenic agents by culture.
• Evaluate effectiveness of chemotherapy, monitor myelosuppression, and evaluate effectiveness of therapy.

Expected Test Outcomes

Some 15 different types of cells in given numbers and stages of maturation are identified.

Test Outcome Deviations

• Leukemia, Hodgkin's disease, multiple myeloma, anemia, agranulocytosis, polycythemia vera, myelofibrosis. Infection, rheumatic fever, mononucleosis, chronic inflammatory disease (and many others).

Procedure

- *Aspiration* withdraws a fluid specimen (0.5 mL) that contains suspended marrow pustule from the bone marrow. During *needle* biopsy, a core of actual marrow cells (not fluid) is removed. A small incision is made prior to introduction of special needle. Tape a fresh, sterile dressing to puncture site and apply pressure to the site until bleeding ceases (approximately 5 minutes).
- Label specimen properly and promptly deliver it to laboratory. Document appropriate information in health care record.

Nursing Role

Use nursing process model following pre, intra-, and posttest care guidelines in Chapter 1. See page 8 for list of appropriate nursing diagnoses.

Nursing Diagnosis

- Knowledge deficit related to lack of information or misinterpretation of information provided about purpose and procedure preparation.
- Anxiety and fear related to bone marrow aspiration/biopsy.
- Discomfort or pain related to procedure.
- High risk for injury or bleeding following bone marrow aspiration/biopsy.

Pretest Care

- Sites used for bone marrow aspiration or biopsy will affect precare, intracare and postcare. Sites used include posterior superior iliac crest; anterior iliac crest (if patient is very obese); sternum (not used as often with children because cavity is too shallow; danger of mediastinal and cardiac perforation is too great, and observation of procedure is associated with apprehension and lack of cooperation); vertebral spinous processes T10 through L4 and ribs; tibia (often in children); and ribs.

••••••••••••
CLINICAL ALERT
◊ Before the procedure, obtain a signed legal consent.
••••••••••••

- Assess for contraindications as in severe bleeding disorders (hemophilia).

- Instruct patient about procedure and purpose. Because bone marrow is major site of blood formation, specimens and biopsies provide diagnostic information about many blood disorders. Reassure patient that analgesics or sedatives will be available if needed. Iliac crest biopsies or aspirations may be especially uncomfortable. Offering patient a pillow to squeeze may be helpful.

Intratest Care

- Position according to site selected; and assist in preparing local anesthetic (procaine or lidocaine) for injection, as patient experiences pressure, some pain or "burning" during this process.

Posttest Care

- Monitor vital signs until stable and assess site for excess drainage or bleeding.
- Evaluate discomfort. Administer analgesics or sedatives as necessary. Slight soreness at puncture site area for 3–4 days after procedure is normal. Continued pain may indicate a fracture. Normal activities may usually be resumed after 30 minutes of rest.
- Osteomyelitis or injury to the heart or great vessels is rare but can occur in a sternal site. Fever, headache, unusual pain, or tissue redness or abscess at biopsy site may indicate infection (may be a later event). Instruct patient to report unusual symptoms to physician immediately.
- Remove the dressing in 24 hours.

Bone Scan (TMJ Scan)   Nuclear Medicine Scan Imaging

This test using a bone-seeking radiopharmaceutical is done to image the skeletal system.

Indications

- Evaluate unexplained skeletal pain, assess osteomyelitis and diagnose early skeletal inflammatory disorders, and determine bone viability.
- Stage malignant disease and evaluation of patients with primary bone tumors, fractures and compression fractures of the vertebra column.
- Confirm temporomandibular joint (TMJ) derangement.

Expected Test Outcomes

- No areas of greater or lesser concentration of radioactive material in bones.

Test Outcome Deviations

- Any process enhancing an increased calcium excretion rate will be reflected by an increased uptake finding in the bones; very early bone disease and healing, metastic bone disease, and TMJ displacement and deformity.

Interfering Factors

- False negative bone scans occur in multiple myeloma of bone and follicular thyroid cancer.

Procedure for Bone Scan

- Radioactive ^{99m}Tc phosphate is injected intravenously.
- A 2–3 hour waiting period is necessary for the radiopharmaceutical to concentrate in the bone. During this time, the patient drinks four to six glasses of water.
- Before scan begins, patient urinates, because a full bladder will mask pelvic bones. The scan takes about 30–60 minutes to complete.

Procedure for TMJ Bone Scan

- A radionuclide ^{99m}Tc phosphate is injected intravenously and scanning begins 3 hours after administration. Patient must remain immobile for 21 minutes while detector rotates around the person.

Nursing Role

Use nursing process model following pre-, intra-, and posttest care guidelines in Chapter 1. See page 8 for list of appropriate nursing diagnoses.

Nursing Diagnosis

- Knowledge deficit related to lack or misinterpretation of information provided about purpose and procedure.
- High risk of injury, infection, or radiation hazard related to radioactive pharmaceutical injection.
- Anxiety related to nuclear scan procedure.

Pretest Care

- Obtain and record accurate patient weight.

- Instruct patient about purpose and procedure of test and patient's involvement. Alleviate any fears concerning procedure. Advise patient that frequent drinking and activity in first 6 hours help to reduce excess radiation to bladder and gonads. Assess for incontinence and/or urine elimination problems and notify testing department if there are potential problems.
- The patient can be up and about during the waiting period.
- If patient is in pain or debilitated, assist him or her to void before the test. Otherwise, advise about emptying the bladder before the test.
- A sedative should be ordered and administered to any patient who will have difficulty lying quietly during the scanning period.
- Test should be deferred in pregnant or breastfeeding women.

Intratest Care

- Take care to avoid urine contamination of the patient, patient's clothing, or imaging table/bedding. Patient must lie still during the exam.

Posttest Care

- Assess patient outcomes and counsel regarding possible need for repeat bone scans. The flare phenomenon occurs in patients with metastatic disease who are receiving a new therapy. It is due to a healing response in prostate and breast cancer within the first few months of a new treatment. These lesions should show marked improvement on scans 3–4 months later.
- Urge fluids and frequent bladder emptying to promote excretion of radionuclide.
- Monitor injection site for signs of infection.
- Dispose of body fluids and excretion in routine ways unless patient is also receiving therapeutic doses of radiopharmaceuticals to treat disease.
- Advise pregnant staff and visitors to avoid prolonged contact for 24–48 hours after radioactive administration.

Brain Scan   Nuclear Medicine Scan Imaging

This test using an iodine radiopharmaceutical that crosses the blood-brain barrier is done to image the brain.

Indications

- Evaluate stroke, dementia, abscess, Alzheimer's, epilepsy, Parkinson's, and schizophrenia.
- Detect brain trauma and tumors.

Expected Test Outcomes

- Normal extracranial and intracranial blood flow, normal distribution and symmetry with highest uptake in the gray matter, basal ganglia, thalamus, and peripheral cortex. Central white matter and ventricles are usually not seen.

Test Outcome Deviations

- Abnormal radionuclide distribution in brain diseases and mental disorders.
- The cerebral blood flow in the presence of *brain death* will show a very distinct image of no tracer uptake in the anterior or middle cerebral arteries or the cerebral hemisphere along with the presence of uptake in the scalp.

Interfering Factors

- Any patient motion (coughing or leg movement) can alter cerebral alignment.
- Sudden distractions or loud noises can alter the distribution of ^{123}I-Iofetamine.

Procedure

- The radionuclide (Iofetamine or technetium) is injected intravenously and imaging usually begins within a half hour of administration and takes about 1 hour to complete.
- With the patient in the supine position, SPECT images are obtained around the circumference of the head. (See Nuclear Medicine Scans: Overview, re: SPECT).
- With administration of iodopharmaceuticals, some departments require a dark and quiet environment.

Nursing Role

Use nursing process model following pre-, intra-, and posttest care guidelines in Chapter 1. See page 8 for list of appropriate nursing diagnoses.

Nursing Diagnosis

- Knowledge deficit related to lack or misinterpretation of information provided about purpose, procedure, and radiopharmaceutical risk.

- High risk for injury/radioactive hazard related to radio-pharmaceutical injection.
- Anxiety related to any type of brain function test.

Pretest Care

- Explain purpose and procedure. Reassure patient regarding safety of radiopharmaceutical. See alphabetical listing of nuclear scans overview.
- Because precise head alignment is crucial, advise patient to remain quiet and still.
- Obtain a careful neurologic and medication history of MAO inhibitors, prior to testing. ^{123}I-Iofetamine should not be used during or 14 days after administration of MAO inhibitors.

Intratest Care

- Provide support and assure that test is proceeding normally.

Posttest Care

- Evaluate patient outcomes and counsel appropriately.
- Monitor IV injection site for infection or hematoma.
- Routine disposal of body fluids and excretions unless patient is also receiving therapeutic doses of radiopharmaceuticals to treat disease.
- Counsel pregnant staff and visitors to avoid prolonged contact 24–48 hours after radioactive administration.

Breast Ultrasound— Breast Sonogram, Breast Echogram, Sonomammography

Ultrasound Imaging

This noninvasive study is useful for differentiating the nature of breast masses identified by palpation or x-ray mammography.

Indications

- Differentiate a cystic from a solid breast lesion.
- Imaging procedure for male breast, very young, pregnant, augmented, or lactating breast.
- Guidance during biopsy or cyst aspiration.

Expected Test Outcomes

Normal sonographic anatomy of breast tissues.

Test Outcome Deviations

- Presence of space-occupying lesions: cysts, solid masses, hematomas, abscesses, duct dilation, calcifications, lymph metastasis.

Procedure

- A coupling medium, generally a gel, is applied to exposed breast in order to promote transmission of sound. In most laboratories, a hand-held transducer is slowly moved across the breast. On occasion, an automated breast scanner is used which may require patient to assume a prone position with breast immersed in a tank of chlorinated water. The tank contains transducers which are moved by remote control in order to image breast tissue. Total exam time is approximately 15 minutes.

Nursing Role

Use nursing process model following pre-, intra-, and posttest care guidelines in Chapter 1. See page 8 for list of appropriate nursing diagnoses.

Nursing Diagnosis

- Knowledge deficit related to lack of information or possible misinterpretation of information provided about procedure or purpose of exam.
- Anxiety or fear related to perception of diagnostic procedure as frightening or embarrassing.
- Decisional conflict related to test outcome and potential for interventional procedures.

Pretest Care

- Explain exam purpose and procedure. Assure patient that no radiation is employed and that test is painless. Ultrasound can readily discern a breast cyst from a more suspicious solid lesion; since no radiation is used, breast ultrasound is effectively used in very young or pregnant patients.
- If previous x-ray mammograms are available, these should be brought to ultrasound laboratory.
- Explain that a coupling gel will be applied to skin. Although couplant does not stain, advise patient to avoid wearing nonwashable clothing. A two-piece garment is preferred.

Posttest Care
- Remove or instruct patient to remove any residual gel or glue from skin.
- Evaluate patient outcomes, provide support and counseling.

•••••••••••••••
CLINICAL ALERT

◊ Patient must agree to and sign a surgical permit prior to performance of an ultrasound-guided breast biopsy or cyst aspiration.

•••••••••••••••

Bronchoscopy
Endoscopic Imaging

This examination is done to view, diagnose, and treat disorders of the trachea, bronchi, and select bronchioles with a fiberoptic or rigid bronchoscope.

Indications
- Diagnose tumors, determine surgical resectability, and locate site of hemorrhage.
- Evaluate trauma, nerve paralysis, and inflammation.

Expected Test Outcomes
Normal trachea, bronchi, nasopharynx, pharynx, and select peripheral airways.

Test Outcome Deviations
- Abnormal findings indicate fibrosis, cancer, tumors, and signs of nonresectablity, inflammatory and infectious processes.

Procedure
- A local anesthetic is applied to the tongue, pharynx, and epiglottis. Steroids and aminophylline may be administered if the patient is prone to bronchospasms. Bronchoscope is inserted through mouth, nose, endotracheal tube, or tracheostomy and advanced into the pulmonary system.
- Arterial blood gases may be drawn and test values may be altered for several hours. Sputum specimens may be collected for cytology, culture, and sensitivity.
- Continuous pulse oximetry readings indicate levels of oxygen saturation before, during, and after the procedure.

Nursing Role

Use nursing process model following pre-, intra-, and posttest care guidelines in Chapter 1. See page 8 for list of appropriate nursing diagnoses.

Nursing Diagnosis

- Knowledge deficit related to lack of information or possible misinterpretation of information about procedure, equipment, purpose, and preparation.
- Anxiety related to perception of bronchoscopy as frightening and inability to breathe normally.
- High risk for injury related to invasive bronchoscopy.
- Ineffective breathing pattern related to trauma of bronchoscopy.
- Impaired gas exchange related to bronchoscopy.

Pretest Care
··············
CLINICAL ALERTS

◊ Obtain a signed, witnessed consent form.
◊ Ordered lab and diagnostic studies should be completed prior to procedure.
◊ Obtain baseline vital signs.
··············

- Assess for contraindications to procedure: severe hypoxemia or hypocapnia, certain cardiac conditions, bleeding disorders, and severe tracheal stenosis.
- Reinforce information related to purpose, procedure, equipment, and sensations. No pain (lungs do not have pain fibers), anxiety, feelings of suffocation, and dyspnea may be experienced.
- Explain that local anesthetic is bitter and numbness occurs rapidly. Feelings of a thickened tongue and sensation of something in the back of the throat will pass within a few hours. Gag, cough, and swallowing reflexes are blocked.
- Explain NPO restrictions for at least 6 hours pre-procedure to reduce risk of aspiration.
- Instruct patient to remove hairpieces, nail polish, make-up, dentures, jewelry, and contact lenses prior to examination.
- Administer baseline vital signs.

Intratest Care

- Use relaxation techniques to help patient relax and breath

normally during procedure.
- Administer IV conscious sedation as per protocols and watch for untoward reactions.
- Monitor continuous pulse oximetry readings and report low values immediately.
- Collect specimens if ordered.

Posttest Care

- Monitor breathing patterns, lung sounds, and vital signs—have resuscitation equipment and tracheotomy set-up available. Continue pulse oximeter monitoring and O_2 administration if indicated.
- Semi-Fowler's position for conscious patients, side-lying position for sedated or unconscious patients.
- Do *not* administer oral food or fluids until gag reflex returns (about 2 hours posttest).
- Instruct patient to spit out saliva rather than swallow it. Discourage coughing and throat clearing when biopsies have been done.
- Collect sputum specimens as ordered and according to protocols.

··············
CLINICAL ALERTS

◇ Watch for signs and symptoms of bleeding, shock, cardiac arrythmias, allergies, hypoxemia or hypoxia, or respiratory failure.
◇ If fever, tachycardia, and hypotension develop, this may indicate onset of gram-negative sepsis. Blood cultures and aggressive antibiotic therapies, together with other supportive therapies, will usually be instituted.
◇ Laryngospasm or bronchospasm (indicated by respiratory stridor, dyspnea, or wheezing) is an emergency situation. High concentration O_2 administered via mask or positive-pressure ventilation and a calm reassuring manner may suffice to alleviate this condition. If not, racemic epinephrine inhalation, steroids, bronchidilators, muscle relaxants, and intubation may be necessary.
◇ Decreased or absent breath sounds, cyanosis, dyspnea, and sharp pain may indicate pneumothorax and must be treated as an emergency—appropriate measures must be instituted immediately.
··············

C-Reactive Protein (CRP)   Blood

The CRP test is a nonspecific method for evaluating the severity and course of the inflammatory process.

Indications

- Monitor acute inflammation and acute tissue destruction.
- Evaluate progress of rheumatic fever under treatment and evaluate postoperative recovery.

Procedure

- Serum (10 mL) is obtained by venipuncture, following specimen collection guidelines in Chapter 2.

Expected Test Outcomes

CRP: < 0.8 mg/dL

Test Outcome Deviations

- Positive reaction indicates presence of an active inflammatory process.
- Failure of CRP to decrease during postoperative period suggests postoperative infection or tissue necrosis.

Nursing Role

Use nursing process model following pre-, intra-, and posttest care guidelines in Chapter 1. See page 8 for list of appropriate nursing diagnoses.

Nursing Diagnosis

- Knowledge deficit related to lack or misinterpretation of information provided about purpose and procedure.
- High risk of injury, bleeding, hematoma, or infection related to venipuncture.

Pretest Care

- Assess patient's knowledge of test.
- Explain purpose and blood test procedure. No fasting is necessary.

Posttest Care

- Advise patient that repeat testing is done during postoperative period or during treatment for rheumatic fever.

C$_3$ and C$_4$ Complement Component

See Immune Function Tests

CA 19-9

See Tumor Markers

CA 125

See Tumor Markers

Calcitonin

See Tumor Markers

Calcium—Blood and Urine

See Electrolyte Studies

Candida Antibody Test   Blood

This test detects the presence of antibody to *Candida albicans* and is helpful in diagnosis of systemic candida infection which occurs in immunocompromised individuals and can be life-threatening.

Indications

- Evaluate candida infection when diagnosis of systemic infection cannot be shown by culture or tissue sample.
- Evaluate candida infection when positive cultures are obtained from specimens with high potential for contamination, such as urinary tract.

Procedure

- A venous blood sample (7 mL) is drawn.

Expected Test Outcomes

Negative for presence of candida infection.

Test Outcome Deviations

- A titer greater than 1:8 in latex agglutination is indicative of systemic infection.

• A fourfold rise in titer of paired blood samples 10–14 days apart indicates acute infection.

Interfering Factors

• Approximately 25% of the normal population tests positive.
• Cross-reaction can occur in cryptococcosis and tuberculosis.
• Positive results can be obtained with superficial mucocutaneous candidiasis or severe vaginitis.
• Immunocompromised patients frequently give false negative results because of their impaired ability to produce antibody.

Nursing Role

Use nursing process model following pre-, intra-, and posttest care guidelines in Chapter 1. See page 8 for list of appropriate nursing diagnoses.

Nursing Diagnosis

• Knowledge deficit related to lack or misinterpretation of information provided about purpose, procedure, and need for repeat testing.
• High risk of infection or injury related to venipuncture.

Pretest Care

• Assess patient's knowledge of test and clinical history.
• Explain purpose and blood test procedure. No fasting is required.

Posttest Care

• Evaluate patient outcome and counsel appropriately. Check venipuncture sites for signs of infection.
• Advise patient that additional procedures such as repeat blood tests or cultures may be required to confirm diagnosis of an infection with candida.

Carcinoembryonic Antigen (CEA)

See Tumor Markers

Cardiac Catheterization—Heart Catheterization, Angiography, Angiocardiography, Coronary Arteriography

X-Ray Imaging with Contrast

This method of x-ray study views and detects abnormalities in the cardiac chambers, valves, and vasculature by means of invasive arterial and venous catheters which carry contrast media to the right and left sides of the heart.

Indications

- Evaluate and diagnose the type and severity of heart disease, the extent of damage, congenital abnormalities, blood flow, identify cardiac structure and function prior to surgery, and response to therapy.
- Measure pressure gradients, cardiac output, ejection fractions, O_2 content, and O_2 saturation.
- Evaluate angina, other types of chest pain, syncope, abnormal resting or exercise EKGs, symptomatic post-revascularization, coronary insufficiency, ventricular aneurysm, and cardiac neurosis.
- During acute myocardial infarction episode (patient can be sent to surgery immediately postprocedure).
- Therapeutic interventions such as pacemaker insertion.

Expected Test Outcomes

- Normal heart function and structure.
- Normal valves and coronary arteries.
- Normal hemodynamic study results (pressures, cardiac output, ejection fractions), oxygen (normal ejection fraction = >55%).

Test Outcome Deviations

- Abnormal pressures in the heart, great vessels, and between chambers indicate valvular stenosis or insufficiency, ventricular failure, idiopathic hypertrophic subaortic stenosis (IHHS).
- Abnormal blood O_2 studies indicate shunting (congenital or acquired), septal defects, leaks, or abnormal sequence of blood circulation.
- Aneurysm or enlargement, stenosis, altered contractility, tumors, constriction.

Interfering Factors

- Benefits of procedure *usually* must outweigh risks to patient. Some possible contraindications include severe heart failure, severe renal disease, recent myocardial infarction, digitalis toxicity, recent subacute bacterial endocarditis, uncontrolled dysrhythmias, bundle branch block, fever, or marked obesity. However, certain situations may necessitate the procedure, even though risk is greater than normal.

Procedure

- Patient lies on an x-ray table which will be tilted at various angles during the procedure to permit better visualization.
- The catheter insertion site is injected with local anesthetic before catheter insertion. For right heart catheterization, the medial cubital or brachial vein is usually used. The catheter is threaded through the superior vena cava to the right atrium, through the tricuspid valve and right ventricle to the pulmonary artery. Pressure measurements and O_2 saturations are taken from these areas as the catheter is manipulated. NOTE: If left-to-right shunt is suspected, blood samples are also obtained from the superior and inferior vena cava.
- For left heart catheterization, patient is heparinized. Catheter is then threaded through femoral or brachial artery and on through aortic valve to left ventricle. Again, pressure readings are taken. Introduction of contrast material, if done, provides data about left ventricular contractility, contour, size, and presence of mitral regurgitation. NOTE: Left atrial function and measurements are usually calculated from other measurements. If direct measurements are necessary, a transeptal approach must be done by advancing the catheter through saphenous leg vein into right atrium and then passing a needle through catheter in order to puncture atrial septum so that direct pressure readings may be obtained. Patient may be asked to exercise during procedure to evaluate consistent changes (atrial pacing may be done during the procedure in order to stress and rest the heart for those patients unable to move normally; ex: paraplegic patient).
- After catheter is removed, direct pressure is applied to arterial site for approximately 15 minutes. Less time and pressure may be required for venous sites. Protamine sulfate is given to reverse effects of heparinization.
- Icebags and sandbags may be applied over site dressings to reduce risk of hematoma or bleeding. For the same reason, the catheterized extremity may be immobilized to reduce movement.

Nursing Role

Use nursing process model following pre-, intra-, and posttest care guidelines in Chapter 1. See page 8 for list of appropriate nursing diagnoses.

Nursing Diagnosis

- Knowledge deficit related to lack or misinterpretation of information provided about purpose and procedure.
- Anxiety related to potential for risks of procedure.
- Self-care deficit related to inability to tolerate exertion demanded for self-care activities postprocedure.
- High risk for injury or infection related to contrast medium administration.

Pretest Care

- Explain purpose and procedure of test. Assess patient's and significant others' need for knowledge and response to forthcoming procedure. Extensive teaching may be necessary. Describe sensations patient will feel; ie, "pressure" with catheter insertion, transient "hot flashes" with injection of contrast medium, nausea, vomiting, headache, or cough. Explain that sedation may be used but that patient will need to follow directions. Emphasize that chest pain needs to be reported promptly so that medication to relieve pain may be administered.

....
CLINICAL ALERT

- ◇ Obtain a valid, properly signed and witnessed consent form.
- ◇ Assess allergies and anticoagulant status. NPO for 6–12 hours prior to procedure unless otherwise ordered. Check if medication should be given. Patient should void immediately preprocedure. (Diuretics may be postponed until postprocedure.) Check vital signs.
- ◇ See Appendix A for standards regarding contrast media precautions.
....

Intratest Care

- Explain that strapping patient to table is necessary because of tilting maneuvers during test. Provide sedation as necessary, if ordered. Orient to fluoroscopy. Reassure patient frequently. Warn of impending noises, sensations, and maneuvers.

Posttest Care

- Check vital signs frequently, including temperature. Monitor for bleeding or hematoma.
- Assess neurovascular status of catheterized extremities frequently.
- Provide emotional support. Administer pain medication as needed, if ordered.
- Do not take blood pressure in arm used for catheterization. A blood pressure 20% below baseline level needs reporting.

··············
CLINICAL ALERTS

◊ Monitor for several complications. These include MI, arrhythmias, cardiac tamponade, infection, pulmonary edema, hypovolemia, spasm, hematoma or bleeding at cath site, allergic reaction to contrast medium, embolus, thrombus, cerebrovascular accident, thrombophlebitis, pulmonary embolus, or vagal response.

◊ Typical signs and symptoms include pain, dysrhythmias, diaphoresis, anxiety and restlessness, fever, cyanosis, thready or absent pulses, tachycardia, bradycardia, hypotension, chills, change in level of consciousness, abnormal cardiac sounds and lung sounds, tachypnea, hypertension, frothy sputum, swelling, hives, itching, decreased or increased urine output, change in skin color and skin warmth, and paresthesias or paralysis. Prompt notification of physician and rapid treatment may prevent more severe complications.

◊ A bruised appearance around cath site is quite normal. However, swelling or "lumps" should be promptly reported to physician.

··············

Cardiac Enzyme   Blood
Cardiac Injury Studies

Aspartate Amino Transferase (AST) or Serum Glutamic-
Oxaloacetic Transaminase (SGOT);
Creatinine Phosphokinase (CPK, CP) or Creatinine Kinase (CK)
and Isoenzymes; Lactic Acid Dehydrogenase (LD, LDH);
Electrophoresis of LDH (LD) Isoenzymes

Enzyme studies are usually a series of tests done for differential diagnosis of cardiac diseases.

Indications

- Diagnose acute myocardial infarction (MI) and severity of disease.
- Differential diagnosis of other cardiac, liver, lung, pancreas, kidney, or brain diseases.

Expected Test Outcomes

ASPARTATE AMINO
TRANSFERASE

AST or SGOT

Adult
  Male: 8–20 µ/L;
  Female: 6–18 µ/L (slightly
  lower than male)
Elderly: slightly higher
  than adult.
Children: similar to adult
Newborn/Infant: 4 times
  normal level—15–60 µ/L

CPK Isoenzymes

MM—96–100%
MB—0–4%
BB—0%

CREATININE
PHOSPHOKINASE

CPK or CK; Total CK

Adult/Elderly
  Male: 38–174 µ/L;
  Female: 96–140 µ/L
Children
  Male: 6–11 y—56–185 µ/L;
  12–18 y—25–185 µ/L
  Female: 6–7 y—50–145 µ/L;
  8–14 y—35–145 µ/L;
  15–18 y—96–140 µ/L
Newborn/Infant: 68–580 µ/L
Lactic Acid Dehydrogenase: LDH

Total LDH: *Adult*: Normal
range varies considerably
depending on lab procedures.
(A range of 95–200 µ/L; check
with specific lab.)

LDH Isoenzymes

Adult
LDH1   14–26%
LDH2   29–39% Cardiac
       and RBC origin
LDH3   20–26%
LDH4   8–16%
LDH5   6–16% Hepatic and skeletal
Differences of 2%–4% are usually normal

Newborn: 30–1,500 IU/L
Child: 50–150 IU/L

Test Outcome Deviations: AST

- *AST (SGOT) increased levels* in myocardial infarction (4–10 times normal values; peak in 24 hours; return to normal 3–4 days after MI). Severe arrhythmias, severe angina, congestive heart failure with liver damage (10–100 times normal value). Cardiac operations and catheterizations. Also in liver diseases—acute hepatitis, acute cirrhosis, infectious mononucleosis with hepatitis, hepatic necrosis, primary or metastic carcinoma, alcoholic hepatitis, acute pancreatitis, skeletal muscle trauma, hemolytic anemia, brain trauma, necrosis or cerebral infarction, pulmonary emboli, gangrene, primary muscle diseases, severe burns, and crushing injuries.

- *AST decreased levels* in beriberi, azotemia, chronic renal dialysis, diabetic ketoacidosis, and pregnancy.

Interfering Factors, AST

- Exercise may cause increased levels.
- Drugs may cause false positives; antihypertensives, cholinergics, coumarin-type anticoagulants, digitalis, isoniazid, salicylates, narcotics, antibiotics, methyldopa, and contraceptives, vitamins, alcohol ingestion.
- Slight decreases in pregnancy when there is abnormal metabolism of pyridoxine.
- Intramuscular injections.

●●●●●●●●●●●●●●
CLINICAL ALERT

◊ For diagnosis of MI, AST levels should be done on 3 consecutive days because peak is reached in 24 hours and levels are back to normal in 3–4 days.

●●●●●●●●●●●●●●

Test Outcome Deviations: CK, CPK

- *CK or CPK total elevated levels* in myocardial infarction—rises after attack (4–6 hours) and reaches peak several times normal values within 30 hours; level returns to normal 2–3 days after infarction unless new tissue damage occurs.
- *CPK increases* also in acute cerebrovascular accident, progressive muscular dystrophy, ALS, electric shock, cardiac defibrillation, cardiac surgery, thermal or electrical burns, central nervous system trauma, extensive brain infection, delirium tremens and acute alcoholism, polymyositis, hypokalemia, hypothyroidism, acromegaly, and acute psychosis.
- *CPK MM Isoenzyme increases* in muscle trauma, injections, major surgical procedures—MI (may remain elevated 4–5

days after MI), crushing injuries, hypothyroidism, convulsions, and electroshock therapy.

- *CPK MB Isoenzyme increases* in MI (rises in 4–6 hours after MI; not demonstrated after 26–36 hours), myocardial ischemia, Duchenne's muscular dystrophy, polymyositis, dermatomyositis, Reye's syndrome, significant myoglobinuria.
- *CPK BB Isoenzyme increases* in biliary atresia, some heart, small cell, lung, brain and prostatic cancers, metastic cancer, chronic renal failure, pulmonary embolism and infarction, brain injury, subdural hematoma, CVA, and severe shock syndrome.

Interfering Factors, CPK Isoenzymes

- Strenuous exercise (up to 3 times normal); surgical procedure that damages skeletal muscle; athletes have a higher value due to greater muscle mass. IM injections increase levels; childbirth; hypothermia.
- Drugs may cause false positives—decadron, lasix, morphine, anticoagulants, some anesthetics, ampicillin, aspirin, amphotericin B, clofibrate, and carbenicillin.

Test Outcome Deviations: LDH

- *LDH increased* in myocardial infarction—high levels (2–10 times normal) within 12–24 hours and continue for 6–10 days. Pulmonary infarction—increases within 24 hours of pain onset. Other diseases as CVA, hepatic disease, red blood cell disease, skeletal muscular disease and injury, infectious mononucleosis, cancers, acute leukemias, shock with necrosis, heat stroke, pancreatitis, hypotension, intestinal ischemia, and infection.
- *LDH decreased* in a good response to cancer therapy.
- *LDH isoenzymes*: LD1 and LD2 increased in MI, hemolytic anemia, renal infarction. In MI, LD1 becomes greater than LD2. LD3 increased in pulmonary infarction and extensive cancer. LD5 increased in liver disease, and striated muscle trauma and congestive heart failure.

Interfering Factors, LDH

- Strenuous exercise, muscular exertion involved in childbirth, skin diseases will increase levels and hemolysis of red blood cells due to freezing, heating, or shaking blood sample.
- A number of drugs affect levels.

. . . .
CLINICAL ALERT

◊ Because RBCs and kidney cells contain the same isoenzymes as heart muscle, patients with pernicious anemia or renal infarction may have the same serum isoenzyme patterns as those with myocardial infarctions.

◊ In MT, LDH_1 and LDH_2 are "flipped": LDH_1 becomes greater than LDH_2; LDH_2 stays about the same, but the level of LDH_2 increases (due to heart muscle damage and release of enzymes into circulation).
. . . .

Procedure

• Blood (7–10 mL) obtained by venipuncture according to specimen collection guidelines in Chapter 2. Avoid hemolysis.

• Note any drugs patient is taking on lab slip or computer screen. Note if patient is receiving multiple IM injections on lab slip. Record data and time when blood was drawn on lab slip for accurate evaluation of pattern of enzyme elevations. No food or fluid is restricted.

Nursing Role

Use nursing process model following pre-, intra-, and posttest care guidelines in Chapter 1. See page 8 for list of appropriate nursing diagnoses.

Nursing Diagnosis

• Knowledge deficit related to lack or possible misinterpretation of information provided about purpose and procedure for enzyme tests.

• High risk for injury, bleeding, hematoma, or infection related to venipuncture.

• Ineffective individual coping related to test outcome and inability to accept diagnosis, including any limitations that the disease may cause.

Pretest Care

• Explain purpose and procedure of test and venipuncture. Enzymes are present in heart, liver, muscles, brain, and lungs and are released into blood following injury or death of cells. Explain need for frequent venipuncture associated with serial testing of enzymes.

• If possible, hold drugs for 12 hours, with physician approval, that may interfere with test results.

Posttest Care

- Apply pressure or a pressure dressing to the venipuncture site. Monitor venipuncture site for bleeding or infection.
- Relate elevated serum levels to patient's clinical signs and symptoms. Report all elevated enzyme levels to the physician immediately so appropriate medical interventions are not delayed.
- Evaluate patient outcomes and counsel appropriately, ie, if new MI need for life-style adjustment, activity, diet, medications, work and leisure activity. Assess patient's anxiety level—be supportive—assess for symptoms of impending MI, such as chest pain, dyspnea, diaphoresis, clammy skin, pallor, and arrhythmias.

CAT Scan—CT Scan, CT of (Head, Body, Abdomen, Pelvis, Spine, Extremities)

X-Ray Imaging with Contrast

CT is a specialized procedure in which a thin beam of x-rays is directed at and moves around some stationary body part, with resultant computer-manipulated pictures that are not obscured by overlying anatomy.

Indications

- Evaluate head trauma and rule out intracranial lesions, aneurysms, and hydrocephalus.
- Rule out intra-abdominal pathology.

Expected Test Outcomes

No evidence of pathology. Normal size, location, and appearance of structures.

Test Outcome Deviations

- Head CT abnormalities refer to aneurysms, cysts, tumors, abscesses, intracranial hemorrhage, hematomas, hydrocephalus, fractures, and degenerative processes.
- Body CT abnormalities refer to neoplasms, metastases, cysts, enlarged lymph nodes, ascites, organ enlargement, aneurysms, and diffuse changes in liver, kidneys, spleen, and pancreas.

Interfering Factors

• Patient movement will result in suboptimal images.
• Retained barium may obscure visualization of organs in pelvic and abdominal regions.

Procedure for CT of Head

• Patient lies on a motorized couch with head supported in appropriate position. Couch is moved into a donut-shaped gantry which encases x-ray apparatus and detectors. Some dull noise may be noticed by patient as equipment moves about. An intravenous contrast medium injection is usually administered. This may induce mild flushing and/or nausea/vomiting. Multiple images are taken while patient remains motionless. Sedation and analgesics may be ordered if it is difficult for patient to lie quietly. Total exam time is approximately 30–45 minutes.

Procedure for CT of Body/Abdomen

• Same as above with the following exceptions: an oral iodine contrast is consumed prior to exam if upper GI tract is to be examined. An IV iodine contrast is usually administered for other exams. This injection may induce mild flushing and/or nausea and vomiting.
• Modifications to body/abdomen procedure are used when performing a *CT scan of the pelvis*. This procedure, although similar, may involve administration of a contrast enema at time of pelvic CT scan.
• In *CT exams of the spine*, protocol is similar except that CT of spine performed to rule out fractures does not require contrast media administration or preparation. CT of spine for cord and paraspinous evaluation will generally require an intrathecal contrast administration and may be performed in conjunction with a *myelogram*.
• *CT exams of the extremities* may be ordered. No contrast or preparation is required if being performed to evaluate bony detail. Extremity CT scans performed for soft tissue abnormalities will usually require contrast administration.

Nursing Role

Use nursing process model following pre-, intra-, and posttest care guidelines in Chapter 1. See page 8 for list of appropriate nursing diagnoses.

Nursing Diagnosis

- Knowledge deficit related to lack or possible misinterpretation of information provided about procedure or purpose.
- Anxiety and fear related to unfamiliarity with diagnostic procedure and equipment.
- Ineffective coping related to test outcome and inability to accept diagnosis of disease.
- High risk of injury related to administration of iodine contrast.

Pretest Care

- Assess for test contraindications (pregnancy, iodine hypersensitivity), evidence of severe renal impairment (elevated BUN, creatinine), and food/beverage consumed within 4 hours prior to contrast administration.
- Explain exam purpose and procedure. Food and fluid restrictions prior to contrast-enhanced studies are generally indicated. Check with laboratory for specific instructions.
- Reassure patient that claustrophobic fears of being in the machine are common. Show a picture of the scanner.
- See Appendix A for standards regarding contrast media precautions.

Intratest Care

- Observe for evidence of reactions such as nausea, skin rashes, hives. Document and inform physician.

Posttest Care

- Evaluate patient outcomes; provide support and counseling.

Cerebrospinal Fluid Analysis (CSF)   Spinal Fluid

Appearance, Volume, Pressure, Chlorides, Glucose, Proteins, Total Cell Count, Syphilis, Culture

Analysis of fluid, obtained by lumbar or spinal puncture, determines the various properties of CSF as well as any abnormal constituents.

Indications

- Diagnose spinal cord and brain diseases such as meningitis and intracranial hemorrhage.

- Measure level of pressure to determine impairment of CSF flow.
- Lower intracranial pressure by removal of a volume of fluid.

Expected Test Outcomes

Appearance: crystal clear, colorless.
  Volume: 90–150 mL; child: 60–100 mL.
Pressure: 50–180 mm H_2O
Chlorides: 118–132 mEq/L
Total Cell Count: 0–5 WBCs, O-RBCs, < 5 lymphocytes
Glucose: 40–70 mg/dL
Protein: Neonates: 15–100 mg/dL; 3 mo.–6 years: 15–45 mg/dL; > 6 years: 15–45 mg/dL.
Syphilis: VDRL negative.
Culture: Negative; no bacteria or viruses.

Test Outcome Deviations

- *Increased pressure* occurs in intracranial tumors or abscesses, meningitis, inflammatory processes, subarachnoid and cerebral hemorrhage, and subdural hematoma.
- *Decreased pressure* occurs in leaking of spinal fluid, complete subarachnoid bleed, circulatory collapse, and severe dehydration and hyperosmolality.

Interfering Factors, Pressure

- Anxiety, breath holding, abnormal venous compression.
- *Change in color/appearance* in inflammatory diseases, hemorrhage, tumors that bring about an elevated cell count. *Blood evenly mixed in all three tubes* occurs in subarachnoid and cerebral hemorrhage. *Xanthochromia* (pale pink to dark yellow), grading is 1+ to 4+, associated with bilirubin, oxyhemoglobin, methoglobin, increased CSF protein, carotene, and melanoma.

Interfering Factors, Appearance

- Traumatic tap and skin disinfectant cause abnormal color.
- *Chloride decreases* associated with tubercular and bacterial meningitis.

Interfering Factors, Chloride

- Concurrent IV chloride and traumatic tap will invalidate results.
- *Glucose decrease* reflects bacterial activity because all types of organisms consume glucose as in pyogenic, tubercular, and

fungal infections. Occurs in lymphomas and leukemia with meningeal spread and mumps, or meningoencephalitis.

- *Glucose increased levels* associated with diabetes and diabetic coma. *Normal levels* usually found in viral infections of brain and meninges and aseptic meningitis.
- *Proteins increased* with increased permeability of CSF barriers in infections, hemorrhage, endocrine disorders, and metabolic conditions. Associated with obstructions of CSF circulation in tumors and abscesses and in meningitis, Guillain Barré syndrome, multiple sclerosis, neurosyphilis.
- *Proteins decreased* in CSF leakage and volume removal, intracranial hypertension, and hyperthyroidism.

···············
CLINICAL ALERT
Total Cell Count
◊ Normally, CSF is essentially free of cells.
···············

- *WBC increase (pleocytosis)* occurs in inflammation, purulent infections, hemorrhage, neoplasms, and trauma. Also associated with repeated lumbar puncture, pneumoencephalogram, injection of contrast medium anticancer drugs, lumbar puncture contaminated by detergent. Malignant cells found with metastatic brain tumors. Increased plasma cells associated with lymphocytic reactions.

Procedure
- Lumbar puncture sterile procedure is performed by the physician, with nurse assisting and providing supportive care to the patient and collecting of the specimens.
- A local anesthetic is injected after skin is cleansed with an antiseptic solution. A spinal needle with stylet is inserted midline between the spines of the lumbar sac between L4 and L5 or lower (subarachnoid space). Sterile manometer is attached to the needle and the opening CSF pressure is measured and documented and 4 sterile collection tubes are filled with 5–10 mL of CSF.

Nursing Role
Use nursing process model following pre-, intra-, and posttest care guidelines in Chapter 1. See page 8 for list of appropriate nursing diagnoses.

Nursing Diagnosis

- Knowledge deficit related to lack of information or possible misinterpretation of information provided about procedure, equipment, purpose, and preparation.
- Anxiety related to perception of the lumbar puncture procedure as frightening and painful.
- Altered comfort related to test procedure, position, and possible posttest headache.
- High risk of injury and/or infection related to the procedure.

Pretest Care

••••••••••••••
CLINICAL ALERT
◊ Obtain a signed, witnessed consent form if institution requires.
••••••••••••••

- Assess for contraindications to the procedure such as soft tissue or other skin conditions and skin infection of puncture site. Infection processes often increase intracranial pressure. Severe degenerative vertebral joint disease, severe psychiatric problems, and chronic back pain need to be considered.
- Perform a baseline neurologic assessment, including strength, sensation, and movement of the legs and vital signs.
- Explain the purpose, procedure, no fasting necessary, equipment, and sensations—patient may feel the entry ("pop" of the needle through the dura mater) even though an anesthetic is used with the procedure.
- Instruct the patient to empty bladder and bowels prior to the procedure.
- Explain that it is important to lie very still throughout procedure to avoid traumatic injury. Instruct on how to relax, deep breathe slowly, inhaling through the nose and exhaling by mouth.

Intratest Care

- Assist patient throughout test to maintain side-lying position with head flexed onto chest and knees drawn up, but not compressing abdomen (fetal position or lateral decubitus).
- Before the pressure reading is taken, the patient is asked to relax and straighten legs to reduce intraabdominal pressure, which causes increased CSF pressure.
- Label tubes with patient's name, date, room number, and tube number (#1 cell count, #2 culture, #3 protein and glu-

cose, #4 syphilis and other studies in order as taken). Take
the specimens to the laboratory immediately (never refrigerate) for analysis.
- Note any leakage of fluid after test is completed.
- Apply bandage dressing to puncture site.
- Record in patient's record time of procedure, condition and
  reaction of patient, appearance of CSF, pressure readings,
  time specimen sent to lab and tests requested.

••••••••••••
CLINICAL ALERT

◇ If initial pressure is near 200 mm, only 1–2 mL of fluid should
be removed to avoid spinal cord compression or cerebellar
herniation. If initial pressure is normal, the Queckenstedt's
test (application of pressure on both jugular veins to produce
increased CSF pressure) may be done. This test is not done if
a central nervous system tumor is suspected.
••••••••••••

Posttest Care

- Instruct patient to lie prone (flat or horizontal) for at least 2
  hours. Turning from side to side is permitted.
- Headaches are common because of spinal fluid leakage from
  site of lumbar puncture. Administer ordered analgesics for
  these and encourage a longer period of bed rest.
- Assess for neurologic status and changes such as increased
  temperature, increased blood pressure, change in level of
  conscious state, irritability, change in pupil reaction, and
  numbness and tingling sensations in extremities.
- Encourage fluids to help replace lost CSF, thus aiding in prevention or relief of headache.
- Check puncture site frequently for fluid leakage and report
  immediately to physician.
- Counsel patient and family regarding posttest outcomes and
  explain/reinforce outcomes as discussed by physician. Prepare patient for potential altered life-style adjustments that
  may occur as a result of test outcomes that indicate permanent neurologic damage.

Chest Radiography (Chest X-Ray)   X-Ray Imaging

The chest x-ray is a very common procedure used to demonstrate the appearance of the lungs, mediastinum, bony thorax, and cardiac silhouette.

Indications

- Evaluate suspected pulmonary or cardiac disease and trauma to chest.
- Determine location of chest tube, feeding tube, catheters.
- Follow progress of disease.

Expected Test Outcomes

Normal posterior-anterior (PA) and lateral chest radiograph; pulmonary markings, cardiac size; pleura and soft tissue structures, and proper invasive line positioning.

Test Outcome Deviations

- Evidence of masses, abscesses within lungs or mediastinum, pneumonia, pneumothorax, pleural effusion, tuberculosis, cardiac enlargement, and bony changes to thorax.

Interfering Factors

- Optimal chest x-rays require patient to be in an upright position and to hold breath on deep inspiration. Inability to perform these actions may degrade quality of chest x-ray.
- Severe obesity adversely affects image quality.

Procedure

- Clothing is removed to waist. X-rays can penetrate through a hospital gown that does not contain any buttons, pins, or metal snaps. Generally, two views of the chest are taken with patient in an upright position. Sustained full inspiration is required during x-ray procedure. Procedure takes only a few minutes.

Nursing Role

Use nursing process model following pre-, intra-, and posttest care guidelines in Chapter 1. See page 8 for list of appropriate nursing diagnoses.

Nursing Diagnosis

- Knowledge deficit related to lack or possible misinterpretation of information provided about procedure or purpose.
- Ineffective coping related to test outcome and inability to accept diagnosis of chest disease.

Pretest Care

• Explain exam purpose and procedure. Assure patient that test is painless. No preparation is necessary. Make certain that jewelry and metallic objects are removed from chest area.

Intratest Care

• Encourage patient to follow breathing and positional instructions.

Posttest Care

• Evaluate patient outcomes; provide support and counseling.

Chloride

See Electrolytes

Cholecystogram, Oral; Cholecystography

See Gallbladder X-ray

Cholesterol Tests   Blood

*Triglycerides and Lipoproteins, High-Density Lipoprotein [HDL],
Low-Density Lipoprotein [LDL],
Very Low-Density Lipoprotein [VLDL]*

These tests are done to determine disorders of lipid metabolism and to assess risk factors for atherosclerosis and coronary heart disease.

Indications

• Screen for risk factors of atherosclerotic vascular diseases.
• Assess other diseases such as liver, biliary, thyroid, renal, and uncontrolled diabetes mellitus.
• Evaluate effectiveness of diet, medication, and life-style changes (such as exercise) to alter test outcome levels.

Expected Test Outcomes

Cholesterol

Normal values vary with age, diet, and from country to country.

Desirable Range: Cholesterol

Adult: 140–199 mg/dL; child: 2–19 years—90–170 mg/dL; infant: 90–130 mg/dL.

Triglycerides

Values are age-, sex-, and diet-related.

AGE	MALE	FEMALE
Adult (20+)	40–160 mg/dL	35–135 mg/dL
14–20	37–148 mg/dL	39–124 mg/dL
9–14	32–125 mg/dL	37–131 mg/dL
0–9	30–100 mg/dL	35–110 mg/dL

Lipoproteins—High Density Lipoproteins (HDL)

Male: 32–70 mg/dL; *female*: 38–85 mg/dL; *children*: 30–65 mg/dL.

Lipoproteins—Low Density Lipoproteins (LDL)

Adult: < 130 mg/dL; LDL = total cholesterol − HDL − (triglycerides/5).

Very Low-Density Lipoproteins (VLDL)

25%–50% of total cholesterol.

Test Outcome Deviations: Cholesterol

Borderline range: 200–239 mg/dL; *high*: >240 mg/dL.

- *Elevated cholesterol levels* in cardiovascular disease and atherosclerosis, type II familial hypercholesterolemia, idiopathic hypercholesterolemia, obstructive jaundice, biliary cirrhosis, hypothyroidism, von Gierke's disease, pregnancy, uncontrolled diabetes mellitus, other pancreatic disease, chronic nephritis, glomerulosclerosis, and obesity.
- *Decreased cholesterol levels* in malabsorption, starvation, liver disease, severe cell damage, hyperthyroidism, chronic anemia, Tangier disease, and drug therapy such as ACTH and antibiotics.

Interfering Factors, Cholesterol

- Cholesterol is normally slightly elevated in pregnancy.
- Estrogen decreases plasma cholesterol and oophorectomy increases it.
- Drugs that cause decreased levels or false negatives: thyroxine, estrogens, androgens, aspirin, antibiotics (tetracycline

and neomycin), nicotinic acid, heparin, colchicine, MAO inhibitors, allopurinol, bile salts.

- Drugs that may cause increased levels or false positives: oral contraceptives, epinephrine, phenothiazides, vitamins A and D, phenytoin (Dilantin), ACTH, anabolic steroids, β-adrenergic blocking agents, sulfonamide, and thiazide diuretics.

Test Outcome Deviations: Triglycerides

- Increased levels: Types I, IIb, III, IV, and V hyperlipoprotenemias, liver disease, alcoholism, Nephrotic syndrome, renal disease, hypothyroidism, uncontrolled diabetes mellitus, pancreatitis, gout, glycogen storage disease, myocardial infarction (increases may last 1 year), metabolic diseases related to endocrinopathies, von Gierke disease, stress, high carbohydrate diet, and hypertension.
- > 500 mg/dL—hyperthyroidism with some danger of pancreatitis.
- > 1000 mg/dL—when more serious risk of pancreatitis.
- *Decreased levels:* malnutrition, hyperthyroidism, exercise, congenital α-β lipoproteinemia, and malabsorption syndrome.

Interfering Factors, Triglycerides

- Ingestion of fatty meal or alcohol may increase levels.
- Pregnancy may increase levels.
- Drugs that may give false negative or decreased levels: ascorbic acid, clofibrate, phenformin, metformin, asparaginase, and colestipol.
- Drugs that may give false positives or increased levels: estrogen, oral contraceptives, and cholestyramine.

Test Outcome Deviations: HDL

- *HDL increased levels* (above 100 mg) associated with chronic liver disease or chronic intoxication, long-term aerobic exercise or vigorous exercise, and estrogen and birth control pills.
- *Decreased levels* demonstrate increased risk for coronary heart disease, familial high alphalipoproteinemia and hypertriglyceridemia, hypothyroidism, end stage liver disease, diabetes mellitus, obesity, chronic inactivity, uremia, and homozygous Tangier disease.

Interfering Factors

- Smoking and moderate alcohol intake decreases level.
- Iodine contrast substances interfere with test results; recent

weight gain or loss interferes with test results.
- Exercise raises HDL levels; drugs that may increase levels or cause false positives: aspirin, oral contraceptives, phenothiazines, steroids, and sulfonamides.

Test Outcome Deviations: LDL and VLDL Levels

- *Increased LDL*—familial type II hyperlipidemia, familial hypercholesteremia, and secondary causes such as diet high in cholesterol and saturated fat, nephrotic syndrome, chronic renal failure, pregnancy, porphyria, diabetes mellitus, multiple myeloma, steroids, and estrogens.
- *Increased VLDL*—familial type IV hyperlipidemia and secondary causes such as alcoholism, obesity, diabetes mellitus, chronic renal disease, pancreatitis, pregnancy, estrogen, birth control pills, and progestins.
- *Decreased LDL and VLDL*: malnutrition and malabsorption.

Procedure

- Blood (5–10 mL) obtained by venipuncture according to specimen collection guidelines in Chapter 2.
- Note patient's age, sex, and any drugs patient is taking on lab slip or computer screen.
- Fasting blood—restrict food and fluids 12–16 hours prior to drawing blood. If possible, hold medications after conferring with physician. Water may be permitted in small amounts. No alcohol consumed for 24 hours before triglycerides.

Nursing Role

Use nursing process model following pre-, intra-, and posttest care guidelines in Chapter 1. See page 8 for list of appropriate nursing diagnoses.

Nursing Diagnosis

- Knowledge deficit related to lack of information or possible misinterpretation of information provided about purpose and procedure for cholesterol, triglyceride, and lipoprotein tests.
- High risk of injury, bleeding, hematoma, or infection related to venipuncture.
- Ineffective individual coping related to test outcomes and need to alter lifestyle, such as diet, alcohol, smoking, exercise, stress, and medications to control cholesterol, triglyceride, and lipoprotein blood levels.

Pretest Care

- Explain purpose and procedure of test and stress importance of fasting prior to test to avoid false outcomes. If patient breaks fast, notify physician or laboratory.
- Inform patient that dietary indiscretion within previous 2 weeks may influence test results; patient should not drink alcohol 24 hours prior to triglyceride test.
- Withhold medications according to physician directives and as related to each specific test; ie, lipoproteins hold oral contraceptives, estrogen and salicylates.
- Note if patient has had any drastic weight change last few weeks prior to HDL.

· · · · · · · · · · · · · ·
CLINICAL ALERT

◊ Stress and illness affect HDL, ie, myocardial infarction; therefore, testing should be done 2–3 months after illness.
· · · · · · · · · · · · · ·

Posttest Care

- Monitor venipuncture site for bleeding or infection and allow patient to resume pretest diet and medications.
- Evaluate patient outcomes and counsel appropriately; ie, for high cholesterol levels instruct on importance of decreased animal fat, replacing saturated fats with polyunsaturated fats, need for consistent exercise program, and need to maintain appropriate body weight. At least 6 months of dietary therapy should be implemented before initiating drug therapy for lowering cholesterol levels. American Heart Association has excellent resources for healthy diets to lower cholesterol.
- Assess for other coronary heart disease (CHD) risk factors such as male sex, family history, smoking, hypertension, low HDL-cholesterol concentration, diabetes mellitus, history of cerebrovascular accident or occlusive vascular disease, and obesity, and counsel accordingly.
- In screenings, all persons with cholesterol above 200 mg/dL should be referred to their physician for remeasurement and evaluation.
- Because cholesterol and triglyceride levels vary independently, measurement of both values is more meaningful and patients with cholesterol levels above 240 mg/dL should have lipoprotein analysis tests done (lipoprotein analysis = cholesterol, triglyceride, HDL, and LDL). In borderline cho-

lesterol levels (200–239 mg/dL) and definite coronary heart disease (CHD) or two CHD risk factors, lipoprotein analysis should be performed. It is important to compare results of all tests and not base decisions upon results of one-time screening tests only.

Chorionic Gonadotropin–Human Chorionic Gonadotropin (HCG)

See Pregnancy Tests

Coagulation Studies   Blood

Prothrombin Time, Protime (PT), Partial Thromboplastin Time (PTT), Activated Partial Thromboplastin Time (APTT), Thrombin Time (TT), Thrombin Clotting Time (TCT), Bleeding Time

These series of tests measure the clotting mechanisms of the body and identify type and extent of suspected coagulation disorders. Platelet count, size, and shape, which is also done in suspected coagulation cases, is explained under CBC.

Indications

- Screen preoperative patients and others for bleeding risk and coagulation disorders.
- Investigate symptoms of easy bruising, petechiae, GI bleeding, nosebleeds, and heavy menstrual flow.
- Evaluate disseminated intravascular coagulation (DIC).
- Adjust dosage of anticoagulants and monitor streptokinase therapy.

Expected Outcomes

- PT: 10–14 seconds (Therapeutic range for oral anticoagulant therapy is 2.0–2.5 times normal limit. Each laboratory sets own range.)
- TCT: 7.0–12.0 seconds (Norms vary widely. Check your own lab norms.)
- Bleeding time: 2–9.5 minutes forearm (Ivy method)
- PTT: 30–45 sec
- APTT: 21–35 (Best therapeutic range for heparin is 2.0–2.5 times normal limit.)

Test Outcome Deviations

Prothrombin Time, Protime, PT—Manage oral coumadin anticoagulant dose

- *Increased or lengthened PT* in coumadin therapy, vitamin K and prothrombin deficiency, hypofibrinogenemia, DIC, liver disease, malignant neoplasm, and hemorrhagic disease of newborn (among others).

Interfering Factors, PT

- Many drugs cause lengthened or shorter PT.
- Clear and careful venipuncture required, otherwise PT can be shortened.

Thrombin Time, Thrombin Clotting Time (TCT)— Monitor streptokinase and in DIC

- *Increased or prolonged TCT* in abnormalities of fibrinogen, multiple myeloma, uremia, and severe liver disease.
- Heparin therapy.

Bleeding Time Ivy Method—Screen for platelet function disorders

- Increased or prolonged in platelet function disorders, DIC acquired abnormal plasma factors, vascular defects, leukemia, aplastic anemia, and renal failure.
- *Bleeding time either normal or prolonged* in von Willebrand's disorder.

Interfering Factors, Bleeding Time

- Times vary if puncture is not of standard depth, width, and if incision is touched during the test.
- Many drugs and alcohol prolong bleeding time: dextran, streptokinase, and antiinflammatory meds.
- Unreliable in persons with cold hands or edema or cyanosis of extremities.

Partial Thromboplastin Time PTT, APTT

- Both tests detect coagulation disorders and abnormal clotting mechanisms and together detect 95% of coagulation abnormalities.
- *PTT, APTT increased or prolonged* in hemophilia A and B and in von Willebrand's disease, vitamin deficiency, liver disease, lupus erythematosus, and DIC. Also, in heparin therapy.

- *APTT decreased or shortened* occurs in extensive cancer (except when liver is involved, very early DIC, and immediately after acute hemorrhage).

••••••••••••
CLINICAL ALERT
◊ APTT > 100 sec signifies spontaneous bleeding.
◊ See Appendix C for standards of critical (panic) values.
••••••••••••

Procedures for PT, TCT, PTT, APTT

- 7 mL of venous blood is obtained following specimen collection guidelines in Chapter 2. Sodium citrate, anticoagulant, is added to syringe. Put specimen on ice.
- Do not draw from a heparin lock or heparinized catheter.
- Note any drugs patient is taking on lab slip or computer screen.

Procedure for Bleeding Time—Ivy Method

- After cleansing, the skin of ear or forearm is punctured using a sterile device to a uniform depth of 2–3 mm and width of 1 mm. A stopwatch is started and blood is gently blotted every 30 sec. The end point is reached when blood is no longer blotted.
- If puncture site is still bleeding beyond 15 minutes, discontinue test, apply pressure, and contact physician.

Nursing Role

Use nursing process model following pre-, intra-, and posttest care guidelines in Chapter 1. See page 8 for list of appropriate nursing diagnoses.

Nursing Diagnosis

- Knowledge deficit related to lack of or misinterpretation of information provided about purpose and procedure.
- High risk for injury, bleeding, and/or infection related to venipuncture or skin puncture.

Pretest Care

- Obtain a careful drug history and family history of bleeding and thrombosis in persons examined through coagulation studies.
- Explain purpose and procedures. No aspirin or aspirin-con-

taining drugs for at least 7 days before bleeding time test.
- For APTT tests and heparin therapy, explain that testing is done to monitor heparin anticoagulant dosage: baseline before therapy started, 1 hour before scheduled dose, and when there are signs of bleeding during therapy.
- For PT test and coumadin therapy, explain that testing is done to monitor coumadin anticoagulant dosage.
- Counsel regarding self-medication. Many prescriptions and over-the-counter drugs increase or decrease effect of antico-agulants and affect test outcomes. Instruct regarding never to stop or start any drug without physician's permission. Assume that excessive amounts of green, leafy vegetables interfere with test results.

Intratest Care

- Note and record appearance of petechiae after applying tourniquet for venipuncture; an indication of bleeding ten-dency.

Posttest Care

- Evaluate patient outcomes, monitor and counsel appropriately.
- Assess for bleeding when times are prolonged or increased.
- Examine skin for bruises on extremities and parts of body patient cannot easily see. Record bleeding from venipuncture and injection sites, nose, or groin. Estimate blood in vomitus, expectorations, urine, stools, and increased menstrual flow.
- Explain that scar tissue may form at puncture sites for bleed-ing times.

Coccidioidomycosis

See Fungal Antibody and Skin Tests

Cold Agglutinins (Acute and   Blood
Convalescent Studies)

This test measures IgM autoantibodies that cause the aggluti-nation of the patient's own red blood cells at 0–10°C. They can be found in *Mycoplasma pneumoniae* infections (primary atypi-cal pneumonia) as well as certain hemolytic anemias, hepatitis, and cirrhosis.

Indications

- Assess infection with *Mycoplasma pneumoniae* in patients having a respiratory infection.

Expected Test Outcomes

Normal < 1:16.

Test Outcome Deviations

- A titer greater than 1:32 is suggestive of infection with *Mycoplasma pneumoniae*. A rise in titer during the course of illness is more important than a single high titer.

Interfering Factors

- A high titer of cold agglutinins can interfere with type and crossmatch procedure.
- High titers sometimes appear spontaneously in older persons.
- Antibiotic therapy may interfere with development of cold agglutinins.
- Improper transport and processing of specimen may cause false negative results.

Procedure

- Serum (5 mL) obtained by venipuncture according to specimen collection guidelines in Chapter 2 and transported to laboratory at 37°C.
- When transport at 37°C is not possible, specimen should be prewarmed at 37°C for 30 minutes prior to separation of serum from red blood cells.

Nursing Role

Use nursing process model following pre-, intra-, and posttest care guidelines in Chapter 1. See page 8 for list of appropriate nursing diagnoses.

Nursing Diagnosis

- Knowledge deficit related to lack or misinterpretation of information provided about purpose, procedure, and need for repeat testing.
- High risk of injury or infection related to venipuncture.

Pretest Care

- Assess patient's knowledge of test and related clinical history.

- Explain purpose and blood test procedure. Explain that culture of suspected organism is difficult and this test is an important aid in the diagnosis of *Mycoplasma pneumonia*e infection.

Posttest Care

- Evaluate patient outcomes and counsel appropriately.
- Advise patient that repeat testing may be required later in the course of the illness to confirm the diagnosis.

Colonoscopy   Endoscopic Imaging

Colonoscopy is the visual examination of the large intestine from anus to the ileocecal valve by means of a flexible fiberoptic or video colonoscope that can also produce photographs of the area.

Indications

- Evaluate chronic constipation, diarrhea, persistent bleeding, or lower abdominal pain in the absence of definitive findings from proctosigmoidoscopy and barium enema.
- Follow-up for recurrent disease or pathology and monitor effectiveness of treatment.
- Perform biopsies and other treatment procedures.

Expected Test Outcomes

Normal large intestine mucosa from anus to cecum.

Test Outcome Deviations

- Benign or malignant tumors, polyps, ulcerations, inflammatory processes, bleeding sites, colitis, diverticulitis or diverticulosis, strictures, or presence of foreign bodies.

Procedure

- Patient is positioned on left side and draped properly. A well-lubricated colonoscope is inserted through the anus about 12 cm into bowel. (Encourage deep, slow breathing at this time.) Air is introduced into bowel to aid visualization as the scope is advanced. Better visualization occurs as scope is withdrawn.

Nursing Role

Use nursing process model following pre-, intra-, and posttest care guidelines in Chapter 1. See page 8 for list of appropriate nursing diagnoses.

Nursing Diagnosis

- Knowledge deficit related to lack or misinterpretation of information provided about purpose, procedure, and preparation.
- Anxiety related to understanding actual process and outcome of colonoscopy.
- High risk of injury related to instrumentation during testing process.
- Potential for bowel incontinence (temporary) related to preparation protocol.

Pretest Care

· · · · · · · · · · · · ·
CLINICAL ALERT
◊ Obtain a consent form properly signed if required.
· · · · · · · · · · · · ·

- Explain purpose and test procedure and indicate that exam can be fairly lengthy.
- Instruct regarding a clear liquid diet for up to 72 hours prior to exam (according to physician's orders). All food and fluids are held from midnight before exam.
- Follow agency protocols for bowel prep. Laxatives will need to be taken to thoroughly cleanse bowel. These may be started up to 3 days before exam. Magnesium citrate, castor oil, or bisacodyl tablets are commonly ordered. Tap water enemas until clear may be ordered. Oral lavage solutions ("wash-out solutions") that are saline iso-osmotic and isotonic to the bowel are commonly ordered instead of enemas (ex: Go-lytely or Colyte). From 3 to 6 liters of this salt solution are administered as is over a 2–3 1/2 hour time period (about 12 ounces every 10 minutes). Solution may be instilled per nasogastric tube. Laxative effects usually begin within 1 hour. Consumption of this solution is necessary until stool is clear liquid. If more than 6 liters are necessary, notify physician before administering more. Notify physician if patient history of congestive heart failure or renal disease before administering these preparations.
- Explain that urge to defecate and cramping or gas pains are expected sensations. Adverse reactions to solutions may

include nausea, vomiting, bloating, anal irritation, and chills.
Inform patient of this possibility.
* Keep head elevated when colon preparations are given via
nasogastric tube so that aspiration may be prevented. Suction
equipment should be at bedside.

Intratest Care

* Administer IV analgesics, anticholinergics, or glucagon as
ordered. Monitor for respiratory depression, hypotension,
diaphoresis, bradycardia, or changes in mental status. (See
Appendix B for standards for IV conscious sedation.) Coach
patient to deep breathe and relax.
* Take vital signs per protocols. Properly preserve specimens
and transport to lab immediately.

Posttest Care

* Check vital signs per protocols. Patient should rest for several hours; may resume a normal diet when sedation has
worn off. Inform patient that he/she may expel large
amounts of flatus.
* Observe for complications of bowel perforation, hypotension, cardiac or respiratory arrest (can be caused by overse-
dation or vagal stimulation from the instrumentation).

··············
CLINICAL ALERTS

◊ Patients with congestive heart failure or renal failure are at
greater risk for fluid volume overload when prepped with
oral washout solutions.
◊ "Washout" preps are contraindicated in ulcer disease, gastric
outlet obstruction, toxic colitis, megacolon, and less than 20
kg body weight.
◊ Signs of bowel perforation indicate malaise, rectal bleeding,
abdominal pain, distention, and fever.
◊ Aspirin (ASA) and similar products should be discontinued
1 week prior to exam because of potential for bleeding.
◊ Patients who are paralyzed or have a colostomy are prepped
in usual manner.
◊ Antibiotics may be ordered for patients with known valvular heart disease.
◊ Discontinue iron preparations 3–4 days pretest as black, vis-
cous stool may interfere with viewing.
··············

Colposcopy

Colposcopy permits examination of the vagina and cervix by means of a colposcope, a special instrument with a magnifying lens. It is also used to evaluate males for genital lesions from sexually transmitted diseases, condylomata, and human papilloma virus.

Indications

• Evaluate abnormal papanicolaou (PAP) smear, cervicitis, benign, precarcinoma, or carcinomatous lesions of the cervix or vagina, and other abnormal-appearing genital tissues.

Expected Test Outcomes

Normal vagina, cervix, and genital area.

Test Outcome Deviations

• Leukoplakia, abnormal vasculature, dysplasias, and abnormal-appearing tissue classified as punctuation, mosaic, hyperkeratosis, or white epithelium.

Interfering Factors

• Colposcopy cannot accurately detect endocervical lesions.
• Scarring may prevent satisfactory visualization.

Procedure

• The cervix, vagina, or male genital areas are swabbed with 3% acetic acid (improves visibility of epithelial tissue). Mucus must be completely removed. Use of cotton-wool swabs is discouraged because fibers left on cervix interfere with proper visualization.
• The colposcope does not actually enter vagina. Exam begins with a field of white light and decreased magnification and is then switched to a green filter to better see vascular changes. Suspicious lesions are diagrammed, photographed, and biopsied. Cervicography (for early detection of cervical neoplasia and cancer) may be done in conjunction with colposcopy in women. This method allows photographic images of entire cervix to be taken. Cervix is cleansed and 5% acetic acid is swabbed onto area prior to taking photographs. A second set of photos are taken after aqueous iodine is applied to cervix. Finally, an endocervical smear is transferred onto a slide to be evaluated later.

Nursing Role

Use nursing process model following pre-, intra-, and posttest care guidelines in Chapter 1. See page 8 for list of appropriate nursing diagnoses.

Nursing Diagnosis

- Knowledge deficit related to lack or misinterpretation of information provided about purpose and procedure.
- Body image disturbance related to need for exposure during examination.
- Anxiety related to modesty issues, procedure, and/or potential unfavorable diagnosis.
- Altered sexuality patterns related to postprocedure sexual activity requirements.

Pretest Care

- Assess patient's level of knowledge about examination process and procedure, and explain purpose and process. Have patient void prior to exam.

Intratest Care

- Offer reassurance. Explain that some discomfort may be felt if biopsies are taken.
- Assist with paracervical block if used within the procedure. Place specimens in proper preservative and route to appropriate department in timely fashion.

Posttest Care

- Provide sterile saline or water for perineal cleansing—acetic acid may produce a burning sensation. Explain that a small amount of vaginal bleeding or cramping for a few hours is normal—provide vaginal pads for patient's use. An agent such as ibuprofen may relieve cramps. Instruct patient to refrain from sexual intercourse and not to insert any object into vagina per physician's orders (usually 2–7 days).
- If cervicography has been done, tell patient a brown vaginal discharge (from iodine) may persist for a few days. Excessive bleeding, pain, fever, or abnormal vaginal discharge should be reported to physician immediately.

••••••••••••
CLINICAL ALERTS

◇ Vasovagal response may occur—have patient sit for a while before standing.

◊ Complications may include heavy bleeding, infections, or pelvic inflammatory disease.

•••••••••••••

Complete Blood Count (CBC) with Differential (DIFF)

Blood

RBC, HCT, Hgb, MCH, MCHC, WBC, DIFF,
Platelets (PLTS) Bands, Segs, Eos, Basos, Lymphs, Monos

The CBC with differential and platelet count (hemogram) provides information about the hematologic and other body systems through a series of tests that determine the number, variety and percentage, concentrations, and quality of blood cells.

Indications

• Screen in physical examinations and pre-operative evaluations.
• Diagnose anemia, inflammatory conditions, polycythemia, and clotting disorders; and illnesses not directly related to hematology.
• Evaluate prognosis, response to treatment, recovery from anemia, polycythemia, bleeding disorders, and bone marrow failure.

Expected Test Outcomes

AGE	WBC $\times 10^3$	RBC $\times 10^6$	HGB G/DL	HCT %
0–2 wk	9.0–30.0	4.1–6.1	14.5–24.5	44–64
2–8 wk	5.0–21.0	4.0–6.0	12.5–20.5	39–59
2–6 mo	5.0–19.0	3.8–5.6	10.7–17.3	35–49
6 mo–1 y	5.0–19.0	3.8–5.2	9.9–14.5	29–43
1–6 y	5.0–19.0	3.9–5.3	9.5–14.1	30–40
6–16 y	4.8–10.8	4.0–5.2	10.3–14.9	32–42
16–18 y	4.8–10.8	4.2–5.4	11.1–15.7	34–44
> 18 y, male	5.0–10.0	4.5–5.5	14.0–17.46	45–52
>18 y, female	5.0–10.0	4.0–5.0	12.0–16.0	36–48

AGE	MCV FL	MCH PG	MCHC G/DL	PLTS $\times 10^3$
0–2 wk	98–112	34–40	33–37	140–300
2–8 wk		30–36	32–36	
2–6 mo	83–97	27–33	31–35	

Age	MCV fL	MCH pg	MCHC g/dL	PLTS ×10³
6 mo–1 y	73–87	24–30	32–36	
1–6 y	70–84	23–29	31–35	150–450
6–16 y	73–87	24–30	32–36	150–450
16–18 y	75–89	25–31	32–36	
Adult				
> 18 y, male	84–96	27–32	30–35	150–400
> 18 y, female	76–96	27–32	30–35	150–400

Differen- tial Age	Bands %	Segs %	Eos %	Basos %	Lymphs %	Monos %	Metas %
0–1 wk	10–18	32–62	0–2	0–1	26–36	0–6	—
1–2 wk	8–16	19–49	0–4	0–0	38–46	0–9	—
2–4 wk	7–15	14–34	0–3	0–0	43–53	0–9	—
4–8 wk	7–13	15–35	0–3	0–1	41–71	0–7	—
2–6 mo	5–11	15–35	0–3	0–1	42–72	0–6	—
6 mo–1 y	6–12	13–33	0–3	0–0	46–76	0–5	—
1–6 y	5–11	13–33	0–3	0–0	46–76	0–5	—
6–16 y	5–11	32–54	0–3	0–1	27–57	0–5	—
16–18 y	5–11	34–64	0–3	0–1	25–45	0–5	—
> 18 y	3–6	50–62	0–3	0–1	25–40	3–7	0–1

The differential count is expressed in % and is the relative number of each type of leukocyte. The absolute number is obtained by multiplying percentage value of each.

Test Outcome Deviations:
Red Blood Cells (RBCs)/Erythrocytes

- *RBC Erythrocytes decreases* in anemias, in Hodgkin's, multiple myeloma, leukemia, lupus erythematosus, Addison's disease, rheumatic fever, and subacute endocarditis. Decreased plasma volume as in severe burns, shock, persistent vomiting, and untreated intestinal obstruction.
- *RBC increases* in primary polycythemia and secondary polycythemia, as in erythropoietin-secreting tumors and renal disorders.

Interfering Factors, RBCs

- There are many physiological variants that affect outcomes: posture, exercise, age, altitude, pregnancy, and many drugs.

Test Outcome Deviations:
Hematocrit (HCT) Packed Cell Volume

- *HCT Packed Cell Volume (PCV) decreases* are indication of anemia. Hematocrit of 30 or less means that the patient is moderately to severely anemic. Usually, hematocrit parallels the RBC when the cells are of normal size, and when the number of normal-sized RBCs increases, so does the hematocrit. The hematocrit may or may not be reduced immediately after moderate blood loss and immediately after transfusion. HCT may be normal following acute hemorrhage. During recovery phase, the HCT and RBC will drop markedly.

· · · · · · · · · · · · ·
CLINICAL ALERT

◊ Hematocrit of less than 20.0% can lead to cardiac failure and death.
◊ Hematocrit of greater than 60.0% is associated with spontaneous clotting of blood.
· · · · · · · · · · · · ·

- *Hematocrit increases* in polycythemia, increase in the number of RBCs based upon hematocrit and hemoglobin values; occurs in severe dehydration and shock when hemoconcentrations rise considerably.

Interfering Factors, HCT

- Physiological variants affect outcomes: age, sex, and physiologic hydremia of pregnancy.

Test Outcome Deviations: Hemoglobin (Hgb)

- *Hgb decreases* in anemia, hyperthyroidism, liver and kidney disease, cancer, various hemolytic reactions and systemic lupus erythematosus.
- The Hgb and Hct are both high during and immediately after hemorrhage.
- *Hgb increases* in hemoconcentration, burns, polycythemia, chronic obstructive pulmonary disease, and congestive heart failure (not all inclusive).

· · · · · · · · · · · · ·
CLINICAL ALERT

◊ An Hgb value of less than 5.0 g/dL leads to heart failure and death. Hct and Hgb give valuable information in an emergency situation if not interpreted in an isolated fashion but in conjunction with other pertinent laboratory data. An Hgb value of greater than 20.0 g/dL results in hemoconcentration and clogging of capillaries.

◊ See Appendix C for standards of critical (panic) values.

•••••••••••••

Interfering Factors, Hgb

• Physiological variations affect test outcome: high altitude, excessive fluid intake, age, pregnancy, and many drugs.

Test Outcome Deviations: MCV, MCHC, MCH

• *Mean corpuscular volume (MCV) changes*: Macrocytic RBCs, MCV < 80 fL, occur in iron deficiency, excessive iron requirements, pyridoxine-response anemia, thalassemia, lead poisoning, and chronic inflammation. Normocytic RBCs, MCV of 82–98 fL occur following hemorrhage, hemolytic anemia, and anemias due to inadequate blood formation. Macrocytic RBCs, MCV > 98 fL, occur in some anemias: megaloblastic, of pregnancy and inflammation, hemolytic and aplastic, fish tapeworm infestation, liver disease, alcohol intoxication, and following total gastrectomy.

• *Mean corpuscular hemoglobin concentration MCHC decreases* signify that a unit volume of packed RBCs contains less hemoglobin than normal as in iron deficiency microcytic anemias, chronic blood loss anemia, pyridoxine-responsive anemia, and thalassemia.

• *Mean corpuscular hemoglobin concentration MCHC increases* indicate spherocytosis. MCHC is *not* increased in pernicious anemia.

Interfering Factors, MCHC

• High values in newborns and infants. Presence of leukemia, or cold agglutins, may increase levels. MCHC is falsely elevated with high heparin blood concentration.

• *Mean Corpuscular Hemoglobin (MCH) Increases* associated with macrocytic anemia.

• *MCH decreases* associated with microcytic anemia.

Interfering Factors, MCH

• Hyperlipidemia and high heparin concentrations falsely elevate MCH.

- WBC counts greater than 50,000 mm³ falsely elevate the Hgb value and thus falsely elevate the MCH.

Test Outcome Deviations:
White Blood Cell Count (WBCs)

- *White Blood Cell Count (WBCs) increases* (leukocytes) above 10 × 10³/mm³ usually due to an increase of only one type of white cell (increase is given the name of type of cell that shows main increase, as neutrophilic or lymphocytosis). Occurs in acute infection in which the degree of increase of WBCs depends upon severity of infection, age and resistance. Also in leukemia, trauma, tissue necrosis or inflammation, and hemorrhage.
- *WBC decreases* (leukopenia) below 40 × 10³/mm³ due to viral infections, hypersplenism, bone marrow depression due to drugs, radiation, heavy metal intoxication, and primary bone marrow disorders.

••••••••••••••
CLINICAL ALERT

◊ WBCs below 5.0 × 10³/mm³ represents a critical value, is extremely dangerous, and is often fatal. Notify physician immediately.
◊ Take appropriate action by protecting patient from infection by means of reverse isolation and strict emphasis on hand-washing technique.
◊ See Appendix C for standards of critical (panic) values.
••••••••••••••

Interfering Factors, WBCs

- Hourly variation, age, exercise, pain, temperature, and anesthesia affect results.

Test Outcome Deviations: Differential Count

- *Absolute and percent segmented neutrophils (Segs) increased* (neutrophilia) occurs in acute, localized, and general bacterial infections; gout and uremia, poisoning by chemicals and drugs; acute hemorrhage and hemolysis of RBCs; myelogenous leukemia, and tissue necrosis.
- *Abnormal ratio of segmented neutrophils in ratio to band neutrophils.* Normally 1–3% of neutrophils are band (stab) forms or immature forms that multiply quickly in acute infection.

Degenerative shift to left means that in some overwhelming infections there is an increase in band forms with *no* leukocytes (poor prognosis). *Regenerative* shift to left refers to an increase in band forms with leukocytosis (good prognosis in bacterial infections). Shift to right refers to few band cells with increased segmented neutrophils which can occur in liver disease, myoblastic anemia, hemolysis, cancer, allergies, and drugs. Hypersegmentation of neutrophils with no band cells occurs in megaloblastic anemia, pernicious anemia (PA), and chronic morphine addiction.

- *Absolute percent segmented neutrophils decreased* (neutropenia) in acute bacterial infection (poor prognosis), viral infections, rickettsiae disease, some parasitical, blood, aplastic, and pernicious anemia, acute lymphoblastic leukemia, hormonal causes, and anaphylactic shock.

Interfering Factors, Neutrophils

- Physiologic conditions such as stress, excitement, exercise, and obstetric labor increase neutrophils. Steroid administration affects levels for up to 24 hours.
- *Eosinophils increase* (eosinophilia) greater than 5% or more than 500 caused by allergies, hay fever, asthma, parasitic diseases, (especially with tissue invasion), Addison's disease, hypopituitarism, Hodgkin's disease, lymphoma, myeloproliferative disorders, polycythemia, chronic skin infection, immunodeficiency disorders, some infectious and collagen diseases.
- *Eosinophils decrease* (eosinopenia) due to increased adrenal steroid production that accompanies most conditions of bodily stress as in acute infections, congestive heart failure, infections with neutrophilia, and disorders with neutropenia. Eosinophilic myelocytes are found only in leukemia or leukemoid blood pictures.

Interfering Factors, Eosinophils

- Eosinophile count lowest in morning, then rises from noon until after midnight. For repeat tests, do at same time every day. Stressful states as burns, post-op states, obstetric labor (many others) will cause a decreased count. Drugs such as steroids, epinephrine, thyroxine, among others, affect levels.
- *Basophil increases* (basophilia) with granulocytic and baso-

philic leukemia, myeloid metaplasia, and Hodgkin's disease; also in allergy, sinusitis, inflammation, and infection (among others), with a positive correlation between high basophil counts and high concentrations of blood histamines.

- *Basophil decreases* (basopenia) in acute phase of infection, hyperthyroidism, myocardial infarction, bleeding peptic ulcer, following prolonged steroid therapy, and in hereditary basopenia. Presence of mast cells (tissue basophils) normally not in peripheral blood is associated with rheumatoid arthritis, asthma, anaphylactic shock, hypoadrenalism, lymphoma, mast cell leukemia, and macroglobulinemia.

- *Monocytes (monomorphonuclear monocytes) increases* (monocytosis) in monocytive and other leukemias, myeloproliferative disorders, Hodgkin's disease and other lymphomas, recovering state of acute infections and lipid storage disease, some parasitic and rickettsiae diseases, certain bacterial disorders as TB and subacute endocarditis, sarcoidosis, collagen disease, and chronic ulcerative colitis and sprue. Phagocytic monocytes (macrophages) found in small numbers in many conditions.

- Monocyte decreases (monocytopenia) not usually identified with specific diseases but are found in HIV infections, hairy cell leukemia, rheumatoid arthritis, and in prednisone treatment.

- Lymphocytes (monomorphonuclear lymphocytes) increased (lymphocytosis) in lymphocytic leukemia, lymphoma, infectious lymphocytosis (mainly in children), infectious mononucleosis, other viral disorders, and some bacterial diseases; also in serum sickness, drug hypersensitivity, Crohn's disease, and ulcerative colitis.

- Lymphocyte decreases (lymphopenia) in chemotherapy, radiation treatment, steroid administration, and increased loss via GI tract; also in aplastic anemia, Hodgkin's disease, other malignancies, AIDS, immune system dysfunction and congenital immunodeficiencies.

Test Outcome Deviations: Platelets

- *Platelets (PLTS) increases* (thrombocythemia) over 1 million in malignancies, polycythemia vera, primary thrombocytosis, rheumatoid arthritis, acute infections and inflammatory disease; also in iron deficiency and post-hemorrhagic anemia, heart disease, and recovery from bone marrow suppression.

- *Thrombocyte decreases* (thrombocytopenia) in toxic effects of many drugs, bone marrow lesions, during chemotherapy, radiation, and allergic conditions; also in idiopathic thrombocytopenia purpura (ITP), pernicious, aplastic, and hemolytic anemias, dilution effect of blood transfusion, and viral infections.

Interfering Factors, PLTS

- Physiological factors: high altitudes, strenuous exercise, excitement, premenstrual, and post-partum affect test outcome.

．．．．．．．．．．．．．．
CLINICAL ALERT

◇ A critical decrease in platelet value of less than 20,000 mm³ is associated with a tendency to spontaneous bleeding, prolonged bleeding time, petechiae and ecchymosis. Notify physician and take appropriate action. With an extremely elevated platelet count of 1 million mm³, in a myeloproliferative disorder, there may be bleeding because of abnormal platelet function.
．．．．．．．．．．．．．．

Procedure

- Blood (7–10 mL) obtained by venipuncture according to specimen collection guidelines in Chapter 2.
- Note any drugs the patient is taking on lab slip or computer screen.

Nursing Role

Use nursing process model following pre-, intra-, and posttest care guidelines in Chapter 1. See page 8 for list of appropriate nursing diagnoses.

Nursing Diagnosis

- Knowledge deficit related to lack or misinterpretation of information provided about purpose and procedure of CBC with differential and platelet count.
- High risk for injury, bleeding, hematoma, or infection related to venipuncture.
- Ineffective individual coping related to test outcome and inability to accept diagnosis of serious disease.

Pretest Care

- Explain purpose and procedure. No fasting is required.

Posttest Care

- Monitor venipuncture sites for signs of bleeding or infection.

- Evaluate patient outcomes and counsel appropriately for anemia, risk of infection, and related blood disorders. Monitor patients with serious platelet defects for signs and symptoms of gastrointestinal bleeding, hemolysis, hematuria, petechiae, vaginal bleeding, epistaxis, and bleeding from gums.
- Monitor patients with prolonged severe decreased WBCs for signs and symptoms of infections. Often, such patients will only have a fever. In severe granulocytopenia, give no fresh fruits or vegetables, use minimal bacteria or commercially sterile diet, no IM injections, no rectal temperatures, no rectal suppositories, and no aspirin or nonsteroidal antiinflammatory drugs.

Coombs' Test

See Blood Groups and Types

Cortisol (Hydrocortisone), Cortisol Stimulation/ Cortrosyn Stimulation, Cortisol Suppression Test (Dexamethasone Suppression Test; DST)

See Adrenal Function Tests

Creatine Phosphokinase (CPK), Creatine Kinase (CK) and Isoenzymes

See Cardiac Enzymes

Creatinine

See Kidney Function Tests

Creatinine/ Creatinine Clearance

Timed Urine with Blood

This test (equivalent to the glomerular filtration rate [GFR] measures the rate at which creatinine is cleared from the blood by the kidney; is co-ordered with virtually every quantitative urine test, and measured along with other urinary constituents to assess the accuracy of the collection.

Indications

- Assess kidney function, primarily glomerular function.

Expected Test Outcomes

Urine creatinine: *Men*: 0.6–1.8 g/24 h; *women*: 0.6–1.6 g/24 h.
Creatinine clearance: mL/min/1.73 sqn

AGE	MALES	FEMALES
<20	88–146	81–134
20–30	88–146	81–134
30–40	82–140	75–128
40–50	75–133	69–122
50–60	68–126	64–116
60–70	61–120	58–110
70–80	55–113	52–105

Test Outcome Deviations

- *Increased levels* present in hypothyroidism, hypertension, pregnancy, exercise, congestive heart failure, acute myocardial infarction, diabetic neuropathy, lupus erythematosus, cancers, acute and chronic renal failure, diet (meats elevate level).
- *Decreased levels* present in hyperthyroidism, amyotrophic lateral sclerosis (ALS), progressive muscular dystrophy.

Interfering Factors

- Drugs which cause false positives include antibiotics (cephalosporins, ganamycin, aminoglycosides), L-dopa, methyldopa (Aldomet), ascorbic acid, steroids, lithium carbonate, cefoxitin.
- Drugs which cause false negatives include phenacetin, steroids, thiazides.
- Strenuous exercise affects.

Procedure

- Collect urine in clean container for either 12 or 24 hours. Refrigeration is required. See specimen collection guidelines and standards for handling in Chapter 2.
- A venous blood sample (7 mL) for serum creatinine is obtained the morning of the day that the 12-hour or 24-hour collection will be completed.
- See Appendix E for standards of timed urine collection.

Nursing Role

Use nursing process model following pre-, intra-, and posttest care guidelines in Chapter 1. See page 8 for list of appropriate nursing diagnoses.

Nursing Diagnosis

- Knowledge deficit related to lack or misinterpretation of information provided about purpose and procedure.
- Anxiety and fear related to test outcome and possible need for further treatment.
- Potential for noncompliance related to need for adherence to test protocols.

Pretest Care

- Assess patient compliance and patient knowledge base prior to explaining test purpose and procedure. Instruct patient not to eat meats, poultry, fish, tea, or coffee for 6 hours prior to test.

Intratest Care

- Encourage water intake for good hydration and avoid strenuous exercise. Accurate test results depend upon proper collection, preservation, and labeling. Be sure to include test start and completion times.

Posttest Care

- Evaluate patient outcome. Provide counseling and support as appropriate.

Cross-Match (Compatability Test)

See Blood Groups and Types

Cryptococcosis Antibody

See Fungal Antibody Tests

Cystoscopy (Cystourethroscopy)   Endoscopic Imaging

These examinations are used to view, diagnose, and treat disorders of the interior bladder, urethra, prostatic urethra, and ureteral orifices by means of cystoscopes or cystourethroscopes.

Indications

- Evaluate hematuria and infections (chronic, recurrent, resistant to treatment) and other unexplained urinary symptoms such as dysuria, frequency, urgency, incontinence, or retention.
- Investigate bladder tumors.

Expected Test Outcomes

Normal structure and function of bladder, urethra, ureteral orifices, and male prostate gland.

Test Outcome Deviations

- Abnormal findings indicate prostatic hyperplasia, prostatitis, hypertrophy, polyps, cancer of the bladder, bladder stones, urethral strictures, vesical neck stenosis, fistulas, ureterocele, diverticula, and abnormal bladder capacity.

Procedure

- A local anesthetic is instilled into the urethra 5–10 minutes before passage of the scope. The scope is connected to an irrigation system. Time-frame is 25–50 minutes, depending upon treatment procedures: tissue biopsy, bladder stone crushing, bladder tumor fulguration, and stricture dilatation.

Nursing Role

Use nursing process model following pre-, intra-, and posttest care guidelines in Chapter 1. See page 8 for list of appropriate nursing diagnoses.

Nursing Diagnosis

- Knowledge deficit related to lack of information or possible misinterpretation of information provided about procedure, purpose, and preparation.
- Anxiety and fear related to perception of diagnostic procedure as frightening or embarrassing.
- Powerlessness related to unfamiliar procedure.
- Alteration in comfort related to posttest muscle spasms.
- High risk for injury or infection related to invasive cystoscopy.
- Potential for altered pattern of urinary elimination related to cystoscopy.

• • • • • • • • • • • • •
CLINICAL ALERT

◊ Obtain a signed, witnessed consent form.
• • • • • • • • • • • • •

Pretest Care

• Explain test purpose and procedure. Be sensitive to cultural, social, sexual, and modesty issues. Describe expected sensations—minimal pain or discomfort, a strong desire to void is normal. Emphasize pretest food and drink restrictions. Sometimes, liquids are encouraged to promote urine formation. Liquid breakfast is usually permitted when local anesthetic is used.

Intratest Care

• Administer IV conscious sedation as per protocols. Diazepam (Valium) or midazolam (Versed) may be given IV to relax patient. See Appendix B for standards. Younger men may experience more pain and discomfort than older men. Women usually require less sedation because the female urethra is shorter. Instruct patient to relax abdominal muscles to lessen discomfort. Monitor for side effects such as amnesia.

• • • • • • • • • • • • •
CLINICAL ALERT

◊ Monitor responsiveness and respiratory status. Resuscitation supplies and equipment need to be readily accessible.
• • • • • • • • • • • • •

Posttest Care

• Monitor vital signs frequently in immediate post-exam period.
• Administer medications as ordered (antibiotics and rectal opium suppositories). Make sure patient or family member is instructed regarding prescriptions to be filled.
• Monitor patient (or instruct to self-monitor) about voiding patterns as well as bladder emptying. Evaluate and instruct patient to watch for edema. Edema may cause urinary retention, hesitancy, weak urinary stream, or urinary dribbling up to several days after procedure. Warm sitz baths and mild analgesics may be helpful. In some cases, insertion of an indwelling catheter may be necessary.
• Provide routine or prescribed catheter care if retention or ureteral catheters are placed. Instruct patient/significant other regarding catheter care if patient will be discharged with catheter in place. If urethral dilatation has been done, advise patient to rest and to increase fluid intake.

·············
CLINICAL ALERT

◊ Report heavy bleeding or difficult urination to physician promptly. Sometimes clots form and cause difficulty in voiding. This may occur several days post-procedure.

◊ Assess urinary frequency, dysuria, pink to light-red-wine color, urine and urethral burning—common events after cystoscopy. Progressively more blood in urine is cause for notifying physician.

◊ Monitor for signs of complications. Potential for gram-negative septicemia is present with urologic procedures because the urethra is very vascular and any break in the tissues may allow bacteria to enter the bloodstream directly. Observe for and *promptly* report chills, fever, increasing tachycardia, hypotension, and back pain to physician. Blood cultures are ordered and an aggressive antibiotic regimen is instituted in cases of gram-negative sepsis.
·············

Drug Monitoring

See Panic Values in Appendix C

Duplex Scan Carotid Ultrasound (Duplex Cerebrovascular Sonogram)

Ultrasound Imaging

This noninvasive Doppler procedure provides anatomic and hemodynamic information about the major arteries supplying the brain as an indication of cerebrovascular blood flow.

Indications

• Evaluate symptoms of transient ischemia, headache, dizziness, hemiparesis, paresthesia, language disturbances, and visual disturbances.

• Screen prior to major cardiovascular surgery.

Expected Test Outcomes

Normal vascular anatomy of common carotid artery, internal and external carotids (often vertebral arteries), with no evidence of stenosis or occlusion. Normal blood flow patterns in these major arteries.

Test Outcome Deviations

- Evidence of plaques, stenosis, occlusion, dissection, and aneurysm.
- Carotid body tumor.

Interfering Factors

- Cardiac arrhythmias and disease may cause changes in hemodynamic patterns.

Procedure

- In most cases, patient is asked to lie on an exam table with neck slightly extended and head turned to one side. A coupling agent, generally a gel, is applied to neck. A hand-held transducer is gently moved up and down neck while images of appropriate blood vessels are made.
- During Doppler evaluation, an audible signal representing blood flow can be heard. Both right and left carotid vessels are examined. Exam time is approximately 30–60 minutes.

Nursing Role

Use nursing process model following pre-, intra-, and posttest care guidelines in Chapter 1. See page 8 for list of appropriate nursing diagnoses.

Nursing Diagnosis

- Knowledge deficit related to lack or possible misinterpretation of information provided about procedure and its purpose.
- Ineffective coping related to test outcome and inability to accept diagnosis of vascular disease.
- Decisional conflict related to test outcome and potential for interventional procedures.

Pretest Care

- Explain exam purpose and procedure. Assure patient that no radiation is employed and that no contrast media is injected. Explain that a coupling gel will be applied to skin. Although gel does not stain, advise patient to avoid wearing non-washable clothing.
- Advise patient to remove necklaces and/or earrings prior to exam for safekeeping.

Posttest Care

- Remove or instruct patient to remove any residual gel from skin.

• Evaluate patient outcomes; provide support and counseling.

Electrocardiogram (EKG or ECG) and Signal Averaged Electrocardiogram (SAE)

Special Study

The EKG provides a printed record of electrical activity of a resting heart and chambers (SAE is EKG done at higher frequencies to detect late potentials).

Indications

• Monitor and diagnose heart rhythm disturbances and myocardial ischemia.
• Diagnose systemic diseases that affect the heart, bundle branch block, and axis deviation, and evaluate artificial pacemaker function.
• Determine response to cardiac drugs, effects of electrolyte imbalance (especially potassium and calcium).
• Use SAE to identify persons at risk for malignant ventricular arrhythmias, especially post-myocardial infarction (MI), and diagnose unexplained syncope.

Expected Test Outcomes

• Normal cardiac cycle, consisting of a P wave, QRS complex, and T wave (a V wave may also be observed).
• Normal chamber size and position of heart in chest.
• SAE: No late potentials.

Test Outcome Deviations

• *EKG abnormalities* fall into five categories: (1) heart rhythm, (2) heart rate, (3) axis or position, (4) hypertrophy, (5) infarct/ischemia. Typical abnormalities seen include dysrhythmias, conduction defects, ischemia, infarct, hypertrophies, pulmonary infarct, pericarditis. Potassium, calcium, and magnesium electrolyte imbalance effects, and drug effects.
• *SAE* is positive for presence of late potentials associated with possibility of sustained ventricular tachycardia and sudden death.

Interfering Factors

• *Race*—more common in black population and disappears with maximal effort/exercise. *Food*—high CHO intake. Anx-

iety/hyperventilation—prolonged PR interval, sinus tachycardia, ST depression with possible T-wave inversion. *Deep
respiration*—may shift heart position. *Exercise/movement*—
strenuous exercise before EKG or muscle twitching can affect
waveform. *Anatomic heart position with shift in thorax*—mis-
placement of electrodes and leads. *Ascites, body weight, pregnancy*—can produce left shift in QRS axis. *Birth and infancy*—
right ventricular hypertrophy. *Gender*—women exhibit slight
ST segment depression. *Medication/drug overdose* and *electrolyte imbalance.*
- In SAE, patient movement and talking affects impulse gathering.

Procedure

- Gelled electrodes are placed on the extremities and chest and
attached to the recorder. The right leg is the ground. Six *limb*
leads reflect status of cardiac vertical plane. Six *precordial*
leads provide data about the horizontal plane. Patient's feet
must not touch the bed to prevent leakage that may produce
a distorted recording.
- For SAE, electrodes are applied to abdomen, anterior and
posterior thorax. Several hundred beats are averaged to computer analyze the late potentials.

Nursing Role

Use nursing process model following pre-, intra-, and posttest
care guidelines in Chapter 1. See page 8 for list of appropriate
nursing diagnoses.

Nursing Diagnosis

- Knowledge deficit related to lack of or misinterpretation of
information about EKG procedure.
- Anxiety related to possible diagnosis of cardiac dysfunction
as evidenced by EKG outcome.

Pretest Care

- Explain purpose and procedure of test. Assess cardiac drug
history, other significant cardiac history, and interfering factors. Instruct patient regarding need to remain quiet and to
refrain from talking during test. Shave appropriate areas if
necessary for electrode adherence. Make sure arms and legs
do not touch footboard or siderails.

Posttest Care

- Cleanse electrode sites and equipment used in the test. Patient may resume pretest activities.
- Evaluate patient outcomes and provide emotional support and explanations as needed. Sometimes evidence of prior heart damage is found of which the patient may have been totally unaware.

••••••••••••
CLINICAL ALERTS

◊ EKG does *not* show mechanical state or valvular function. It measures electrical impulses. It may be normal in the presence of heart disease. Conclusions about patient status need to "take in the whole picture" of patient status. An abnormal EKG may not necessarily signify heart disease just as a normal EKG does not always reflect absence of disease. Pacemaker and magnet use should be noted.
••••••••••••

Electroencephalography (EEG)   Special Study

This test measures and records electrical impulses from the cortex of the brain by electrodes attached to the patient's scalp.

Indications

- Diagnose epilepsy, tumors, abscesses, infarcts, injuries, hematomas, cerebrovascular diseases, narcolepsy, tremors, and Alzheimer's; to ascertain brain death ("cerebral silence").

Expected Test Outcomes

- Brain waves have normal symmetric patterns, amplitudes, frequencies, and characteristics—alpha 8–11 Hz (Hertz = cycles per second).

Test Outcome Deviations

- Seizure patterns (grand mal/petit mal) if done during seizure. Focal (psychomotor), infantile myoclonic, and Jacksonian seizures that occur in brain abscesses, gliomas, cerebrovascular accident, dementia, late stages of metabolic diseases, tumors, vascular lesions, metabolic disorders, meningitis, encephalitis, and brain death.

Interfering Factors

- Sedatives, mild hypoglycemia, oily hair/hair spray, artifacts from eye and body movements.

Procedure

- Multiple gelled electrodes are affixed onto the scalp in a definite pattern. The impulses transmitted are magnified at least 1 million times and transcribed to permanent "hardcopy" for further study.
- Patient may be asked to purposely hyperventilate to produce an alkalosis which results in vasoconstriction. This may activate a seizure pattern. Photic stimulation, use of flashing lights over the face at 1–30 times per second, may produce an abnormal electrical discharge not normally produced on EEG. Sleep deprivation prior to test may be ordered to promote rest during test. (Abnormalities frequently surface during sleep.)

Nursing Role

Use nursing process model following pre-, intra-, and posttest care guidelines in Chapter 1. See page 8 for list of appropriate nursing diagnoses.

Nursing Diagnosis

- Knowledge deficit related to lack of or misinterpretation of information provided about purpose and procedure of EEG.
- Potential for sleep pattern disturbance related to sleep deprivation if required for test.
- Anxiety related to any type of brain testing and uncertainty of diagnostic findings.

Pretest Care

- Explain purpose and procedure of testing. Reassure patient that test is not painful, does not evaluate thinking processes or intelligence, and does not produce shock sensations. Sleep deprivation may be ordered. A sleep deprivation EEG requires that patient sleep only between midnight and 4 AM. Special instructions may apply to children. Food and smoking are permitted. Patient should not skip meals. Hypoglycemia alters waves. However, coffee, tea, colas, and other caffeine products should be withheld for 8 hours before testing. Shampoo hair the evening before test. Use *only* shampoo.

• Withhold anticonvulsants, tranquilizers, barbiturates, and other sedatives for 24–48 hours prior to testing unless otherwise ordered. Children may need sedation as may adults who cannot sleep.

Intratest Care

• Instruct patient to relax, remain quiet, and close eyes. Promote a relaxed, quiet environment. Note unusual eye movements and body activity since these can alter brain wave patterns. Be alert for seizure activity and provide proper interventions if necessary.

Posttest Care

• Shampoo hair normally; may help to remove gel and adhesive. If sedation was given, promote rest. Safety precautions should be observed. Otherwise, resume normal activities.
• Observe seizure precautions if applicable.
• Resume medications unless ordered otherwise (consult with physician first).
• Emotional support and teaching help patient to adjust to disorders. Explanations of findings and how they relate to behavior may be very helpful.

··············
CLINICAL ALERTS

◊ Hyperventilation may cause transient dizziness or numbness and tingling in hands and feet.
◊ If needle electrodes are used, a "prickling" sensation may be felt.
◊ Abnormal EEGs occur in impaired consciousness—the more profound the change of consciousness, the more abnormal the EEG.
◊ Between seizures, EEG may be normal.
··············

Electrolyte Studies   Blood and Timed Urine

Calcium (Ca), Chloride (Cl), Phosphate (P), Magnesium (Mg), Potassium (K) and Sodium (Na)

This series of tests is done to evaluate electrolyte, fluid, and acid-base balance in the body, and for early detection of potential or actual imbalances so that corrective treatment can be initiated.

Indications

- Measure calcium (Ca) for parathyroid function; Ca metabolism malignancies, bone disorders.
- Obtain chloride (Cl) for inferential value in correction of hypokalemic alkalosis.
- Measure phosphorus (P) for relationship to calcium and parathyroid hormone.
- Use magnesium (Mg) as index of renal function and calcium absorption.
- Assess potassium (K) to identify unsuspected and anticipated potassium imbalances which can be deadly.
- Assess sodium (Na) for renal and adrenal disturbances and acid-base imbalance.

Expected Test Outcomes

Total Calcium Blood

AGE	MG/DL
0–10 d	7.6–10.4
10 d–3 y	8.7–9.8
3–9 y	8.8–10.1
4–11 y	8.9–10.1
11–13 y	8.8–10.6
13–15 y	9.2–10.7
15–18 y	8.9–10.7
Adult	8.4–10.2

Ionized Calcium Blood

Ionized: 1.15–1.35 mmol/L
Adult: 4.4–5.4 mg/dL
Children: 1–18 y: 1.20–1.40 mmol/L
Newborns: 1.10–1.44 mmol/L

Calcium Urine

Adult: 100–300 mg/24 h/average diet or 2.50–7.50 mmol/24 h
50–150 mg/24 h/low-calcium diet or 1.25–3.75 mmol/24 h

Chloride

Adult and Newborn: 98–106 mmol/L

Phosphate

Adult: 2.5–4.5 mg/dL; 1.0–1.5 mmol/L
Children: 4.0–5.4 mg/dL; 1.45–2.09 mmol/L

Magnesium
Adult: 1.8–2.4 mg/dL or 0.65–1.05 mmol/L

Potassium: Blood
3.5–5.0 mEq/mL or mmol/L

Potassium: Urine
Broad range: 25–125 mEq/24 h or 25–125 mmol/24 h
Average range: 40–80 mEq/24 h or 40–80 mmol/24 h. Diet dependent.

Sodium: Blood
Premature infant: 132–140 mEq/L
Full-term infant: 133–142 mEq/L
1–16 y: 135–145 mEq/L
Adult: 135–145 mEq/L

Test Outcome Deviations: Calcium
- *Total calcium increased* (hypercalcemia) in hyperparathyroidism, cancers, hyperthyroidism, prolonged immobility, granulomatous disease, renal transplant, excessive vitamin D, milk, and antacids.
- *Total calcium decreased* (hypocalcemia) with reduced albumin levels, hyperphosphatemia, hypoparathyroidism, malabsorption of calcium and vitamin D, alkalosis, acute pancreatitis, diarrhea, vitamin D deficiency.
- *Ionized calcium increased* or hypoparathyroidism, ectopic parathyroid hormone producing tumors, excess vitamin D intake, and some malignancies.
- *Ionized calcium increased* in hyperventilation, bicarbonate administration, acute pancreatitis, diabetic acidosis, sepsis, hyperparathyroidism, vitamin D deficiency, toxic shock, and fat embolism,

Interfering Factors, Calcium
- Many drugs cause increases (thiazide diuretics, dialysis resins, magnesium, calcium supplements), milk intake; decreases (excessive use of laxatives).

Test Outcome Deviations: Chloride
- *Chloride increased* in dehydration, Cushing's, respiratory alkalosis, hyperparathyroidism, diabetes insipidus, renal tubular acidosis.

- *Chloride decreased* in severe vomiting and gastric suction, burns, metabolic alkalosis, salt losing renal disorders, some types of diuretic therapy.

Interfering Factors, Chloride

- Many drugs cause changes in chloride levels and increase after excessive saline infusions.

Test Outcome Deviations: Phosphorus

- *Phosphorus increased* (hyperphosphatemia) in renal insufficiency, severe nephritis, hypoparathyroidism, hypocalcemia, excessive alkali intake, healing fractures, bone tumors, Addison's disease, and acromegaly.
- *Phosphorus decreased* (hypophosphatemia) in hyperparathyroidism, rickets, diabetic coma, hyperinsulinism, liver disease, renal tubular acidoses, continuous IV glucose in nondiabetic (phosphorus follows glucose into the cells), vomiting, and severe malnutrition.
- *Magnesium increased* in renal failure or reduced renal function, diabetic acidosis, hypothyroidism, Addison's disease, after adrenalectomy, and diabetes in elderly.

Test Outcome Deviations: Magnesium

- *Magnesium decreased* in chronic diarrhea, hemodialysis, blood transfusions, chronic renal diseases, hepatic cirrhosis, chronic pancreatitis, abuse of diuretics, hyperaldosteronism, laxatives, hyperthyroidism, hypoparathyroidism, malabsorption, alcoholism, gastric drainage, severe burns, and excessive sweating.

Interfering Factors, Magnesium

- Hemolysis invalidates results.
- Falsely increased in prolonged salicylate therapy, lithium, magnesium antacids, and laxatives, and decreased in a number of drugs (calcium gluconate).

Test Outcome Deviations: Potassium

- *Potassium,* a falling trend time (0.1–0.2 mEq/day) indicates a developing K deficiency. Most frequent K deficiency is GI loss. K depletion in IVs without K supplementation.
- *Potassium decreased* (hypokalemia) in excessive renal excretion, diarrhea, vomiting, excessive spitting and drooling of

saliva, eating disorders, malabsorption, draining wounds, cellular shifts.
- *Potassium increased* (hyperkalemia) in renal failure, interstitial dehydration, cell damage, acidosis, diabetic ketoacidosis, nephritis, tubular disorders, pseudo hypoaldosteronism, sickle cell anemia, and systemic lupus erythematosus.

Interfering Factors, Potassium

- Hemolysis causes up to 5.0% increase in K.
- Glucose administration and licorice decreases value.
- Many drugs interfere with potassium levels. IV potassium penicillin causes hyperkalemia; penicillin sodium causes hypokalemia.

Test Outcome Deviations: Sodium

- *Sodium increases* (hypernatremia) are uncommon but do occur in dehydration, starvation, insufficient water intake, tracheobronchitis, and coma.
- *Sodium decreases* (hyponatremia) reflect a relative excess of body water rather than a low total body sodium. Occurs in severe burns, diarrhea, vomiting, excessive non-electrolyte IVs, kidney and liver disease, edema, large intake of water, Addison's, obstruction and malabsorption, and diuretics.

Interfering Factors, Sodium

- Dietary salt and sodium and many drugs cause increases or decreases.

••••••••••••
CLINICAL ALERT

◊ See Appendix C for standards of critical (panic) values.
••••••••••••

Procedure

- Blood (5–7 mL) obtained by venipuncture according to specimen collection guidelines in Chapter 2. Do not add citrate which gives falsely low outcome. Serum is used for calcium, phosphorus, and magnesium. Serum or heparinized blood for chloride and potassium; heparinized blood for sodium.
- List patient drugs on laboratory slip or computer screen.
- Deliver potassium blood specimens to laboratory for immediate exam.

- For calcium, collect urine for 24 hours in an acid-washed bottle if not ordered with other tests. Urine specimens for calcium, sodium, and potassium may be refrigerated. See timed specimen collection guidelines in Chapter 2 and standards for handling and preservation in Appendix E.
- Note drugs patient is taking on lab slip or computer screen.

Nursing Role

Use nursing process model following pre-, intra-, and posttest care guidelines in Chapter 1. See page 8 for list of appropriate nursing diagnoses.

Nursing Diagnosis

- Knowledge deficit related to lack of or misinterpretations of information provided about purpose and procedure.
- High risk for injury or infection related to venipuncture.
- Potential for noncompliance related to inability to follow specimen collection protocols for timed urine.

Pretest Care

- Assess patient compliance and knowledge base prior to explaining purpose and procedure of testing for electrolyte disorders.
- If electrolyte disorders are suspected, record daily weight, blood pressure, accurate fluid intake and output, skin, tongue, urine, EKG, and neuromuscular changes to supply additional diagnostic data.

Intratest Care

- Food and fluids are permitted and encouraged.
- Accurate test results depend upon proper collection, preservation, and labeling.

Posttest Care

- Evaluate patient outcomes and monitor appropriately for signs of excess or deficient electrolytes.

·············
CLINICAL ALERT

◊ Notify physician and institute appropriate treatment at once for critical or panic levels. See Appendix C for standards for panic problems.

·············

Electromyography (EMG)— Electroneurogram (ENG), Electromyoneurogram

Special Study

Electromyography and electroneurography are performed to detect neuromuscular abnormalities through the use of skin and needle electrodes that measure and record nerve and muscle conduction and electrical activity.

Indications

• Define site and cause of disorders both at spinal cord level and peripheral sites.

Expected Test Outcomes

Normal nerve conduction and muscle action potentials upon insertion of electrodes and needles at rest and during minimum and maximum voluntary muscle contractions. Normal conduction velocity rates.

Test Outcome Deviations

• Diseases or disorders of striated muscle fibers or cell membrane, muscular dystrophy, cell membrane disorders such as myotonia, polymyositis, hypocalcemia, thyrotoxicosis, tetanus, rabies; myasthenia gravis, deficiencies such as familial hypokalemia or McArdle's phosphorylase.
• Carcinomas, hyperadrenocorticism, presence of acetylcholine blockers (curare, botulism, kanamycin, snake venom).
• Disorders of lower motor neuron anterior horn of spinal cord (myelopathy) such as tumors, traumas, syringomyelia, muscular dystrophy, congenital amyotonia, anterior poliomyelitis, ALS, peroneal muscular atrophy. Lesions of nerve root (radioculopathy) such as Guillain-Barré or nerve root entrapment from tumor, trauma, herniated disc, spurs, or stenosis. Peripheral or axial nerve damage from entrapment, endocrine disorders such as hypothyroidism or diabetes, toxins, and peripheral nerve degeneration and regeneration.

Interfering Factors

• Decreased conduction in elderly, pain, extraneous electrical activity, edema, hemorrhage, or thick, subcutaneous fat.

Procedure

- A ground electrode is applied to patient. Patient needs to relax or to contract certain muscle groups.
- There are two parts to the test: when testing for *nerve conduction*, electrical current is passed through an electrode placed over a specific site. Sensations perceived by patient are normally not unpleasant.
- The second test determines *muscle potential*. A needle electrode is inserted into muscle and moved or advanced as needed in order to detect muscle electrical responses. If needle strikes a terminal nerve, patient may experience pain. Contractions of muscles will produce sounds like a machine gun being fired or hail stones on a tin roof.

Nursing Role

Use nursing process model following pre-, intra-, and posttest care guidelines in Chapter 1. See page 8 for list of appropriate nursing diagnoses.

Nursing Diagnosis

- Knowledge deficit related to lack of or possible misinterpretation of information provided about test purpose and procedure.
- Anxiety related to potential for experiencing pain during procedure.
- Discomfort or pain related to EMG or ENG procedures.
- High risk for injury or hematomas related to inability to perceive normal sensations and testing procedures.

Pretest Care

- Explain purpose and procedure of test. Sedation or analgesics may be ordered.

Intratest Care

- Explain procedure as it progresses. Alert patient to possible sensations that may be felt. Instruct patient to inform diagnostician of pain, as this may alter results.

Posttest Care

- Provide pain relief if necessary. Promote rest and relaxation, especially if test has been lengthy.

∙∙∙∙∙∙∙∙∙∙∙∙∙∙
CLINICAL ALERT

◊ Recent anticoagulant therapy may increase risk of bleeding or hematoma during muscle potential testing.

∙∙∙∙∙∙∙∙∙∙∙∙∙∙

Electrophysiology   Special Study
Procedure—EP Studies
Bundle of HIS Procedure

This invasive procedure is done to diagnose and treat ventricular dysrhythmias by measuring the cardiac conduction system through solid lumen (rather than open-lumen) catheters, advanced through the veins to the right atrium and right ventricle.

Indications

• Diagnose conduction system defects and differentiate supraventricular from ventricular rhythms and establish etiologies of disorders, or to "work-up" complaints of syncope or sick sinus syndrome.
• Evaluate drug treatment effectiveness and pace the heart in order to induce certain dysrhythmias during studies.

Expected Test Outcomes

Normal conduction, refractory, and recovery times.

Test Outcome Deviations

• Longer or shorter conduction intervals, longer refractory periods, or prolonged recovery times, induced dysrhythmias, long atria common (HIS) bundle (AH) intervals = A/V node disease in absence of vagal and sympathetic influences, and long common (HIS) bundle ventricle (HV) intervals = HIS-Purkinje system disease.
• Prolonged sinus node recovery time = sinus node dysfunction, sino-atrial conduction times = sinus exit block; HIS bundle split or widening = lesion of bundle of HIS and recurrent ventricular tachycardia able to be induced (confirms diagnosis of recurrent ventricular tachycardia).

Procedure

• Antecubital or groin insertion site is chosen (depends upon location of catheter placement in the heart and condition of the patient's veins). Baseline values are recorded. This may require pacing (eg: to measure sinus node recovery times it may be necessary to perform atrial pacing until the sinus becomes fatigued). Pacing is used to induce arrhythmias. Sustained arrhythmias that are symptomatic may require cardioversion or defibrillation. Continuous conversation with the patient is maintained in order to assess ongoing level of consciousness.

• Sterile pressure dressings are applied to catheter insertion sites postprocedure. Procedure may take several hours, especially with complex arrhythmias.

Nursing Role

Use nursing process model following pre-, intra-, and posttest care guidelines in Chapter 1. See page 8 for list of appropriate nursing diagnoses.

Nursing Diagnosis

• Knowledge deficit related to lack of or misinterpretation of information about EP study purpose and procedure.
• High risk for decreased cardiac output related to induced dysrhythmias during procedure.
• High risk of injury related to potential for cardiac arrest during procedure.

Pretest Care

• Explain purpose and procedure of test. Describe sensations that may be felt such as "crawling" as the catheter is advanced, palpitations, "racing" heart, lightheadedness or dizziness. Emphasize that lightheadedness or dizziness must be reported immediately. Evaluate neuro status for deficits. Patient needs to be NPO for at least 3 hours before procedure and should void immediately before study, if possible. Record baseline vital signs.

••••••••••••
CLINICAL ALERT
◇ Obtain a properly signed and witnessed consent form.
••••••••••••

Intratest Care

• Explain procedure and sensations as procedure progresses. Converse on a continuum to establish level of consciousness.

- Record vital signs per protocols.

Posttest Care

- Flat bedrest for 6–8 hours; no bending of extremities used for catheter introduction is allowed—immobilize as necessary. Uninvolved extremities may be moved or exercised. Sometimes turning to the side is permitted, provided the catheterized extremity remains extended for prescribed period of time.
- Check vital signs, catheter sites, and neurovascular status (color, motion such as wiggling toes, sensation, warmth, capillary refill times, and pulses) per protocols.
- Give analgesics as ordered.
- Should the EP study catheter be left in place for sequential studies, it is sutured in place and covered with sterile dressings. Certain protocols may be ordered for care of this catheter.

············
CLINICAL ALERTS

◊ Drug side effects must be considered and anticipated (eg: hypotension, cramping, venous pain, euphoria).
◊ Resuscitation equipment and drugs should be readily available at all times.
◊ Be alert to possibility of hematoma or bleeding at catheter sites.
············

Endoscopic Retrograde Cholangiopancreatography (ERCP)

Endoscopic and X-ray Imaging with Contrast

The pancreatic ducts and hepatobiliary tree are examined by fiberoptic endoscopy and x-ray.

Indications

- Evaluate jaundice, pancreatitis, abdominal pain, malformations, stenosis, tumors, and other disease processes.
- Perform procedures such as biopsies, calculi removal, dilatations, or drain insertions.

Expected Test Outcomes

Patent normal pancreatic ducts, hepatic ducts, common bile ducts, duodenal papilla, ampulla of Vater, and gallbladder.

Test Outcome Deviations

- Abnormal findings include calculi, stenosis, cirrhosis, fibrosis, primary sclerosing cholangitis, cysts, pseudocysts, tumors, or pancreatitis.

Procedure

- If barium studies have preceded ERCP, a KUB x-ray should be done to check for residual barium that may obscure views during ERCP. An IV line to be used for IV sedation and other drugs is started before the procedure. Patient's throat is numbed with a topical anesthetic spray or gargle. Patient is placed in left lateral position with knees flexed (as endoscope is inserted through a mouthpiece) and changed to prone position when instructed to do so. Simethicone may be instilled to reduce bubbling from bile. Glucagon or anticholinergics may be given IV to relax duodenum so papilla can be cannulated.
- Iodine contrast is instilled to outline pancreatic and common bile ducts after the ampulla of Vater is cannulated. Fluoroscopy and x-ray studies are done at this time.

Nursing Role

Use nursing process model following pre-, intra-, and posttest care guidelines in Chapter 1. See page 8 for list of appropriate nursing diagnoses.

Nursing Diagnosis

- Knowledge deficit related to lack of or misinterpretation of information provided about purpose and procedure of test.
- Anxiety related to actual testing procedure and test outcomes.
- Discomfort related to ERCP procedure.
- High risk for impaired ventilation related to actual procedure or positioning.

Pretest Care

- Explain purpose and procedure of ERCP. Emphasize that procedure can be lengthy and that certain sensations, such as difficulty swallowing (from local anesthetic), drowsiness, dry mouth together with thirst, tachycardia, urine retention, or blurring of vision (from anticholinergics), may be present. Glucagon may produce nausea, vomiting, hives, or flushing. Contrast medium may also cause transient flushing. See Appendix A for standards regarding contrast media precautions.

•••••••••••••
CLINICAL ALERT

◇ Obtain properly signed and witnessed consent form.
•••••••••••••

- Remove jewelry, contact lenses, dentures, and store safely.
- Ascertain that patient has been NPO since midnight. Check for allergies to medications, iodine, and contrast media. Evaluate lab results and other studies. Inform physician of abnormal values or results. Evaluate patient's health status relative to complaints of pain, respiratory difficulty, bleeding, or other significant events. Obtain baseline vital signs. Patient should void pre-procedure (urine retention can occur after anticholinergics).
- Explain that patient should swallow when instructed to do so, that choking sensations are normal, that patient will have to lie quietly during x-rays, and that deep breathing may relieve gagging.

Intratest Care

- Insert mouthpiece. Explain that oral suctioning may be necessary. Reposition patient and administer medications as requested by physician. Monitor patient's respiratory and cardiac status. Properly label specimens and route to appropriate department in a timely manner. See Appendix B for standards regarding IV conscious sedation.

Posttest Care

- Monitor vital signs including temperature and assess for effects of IV sedation and other medications. Observe respiratory status. Withhold fluids and food until gag reflex returns (about 2 hours). Reassure patient that sore throat and abdominal discomfort may persist for several hours.
- Make sure that patient voids within 8 hours postprocedure.
- Instruct patient not to perform tasks that require mental alertness or to sign legal documents for 24 hours.
- Gargles, oral fluids, or lozenges can soothe a sore throat.

•••••••••••••
CLINICAL ALERTS

◇ Have resuscitation equipment readily accessible. Mazicon and naloxone should be available to reverse sedation effects if necessary. Notify physician of pain with swallowing or neck movement, substernal or epigastric pain worsened with breathing or movement, hypotension, shoulder pain, dyspnea, abdominal or back pain, cyanosis, fever, chills, or left-upper quadrant pain or tenderness. These symptoms may signal complications such as perforation, cholangitis, pancreatitis, or gram-negative septicemia.

••••••••••••••

Eosinophils

See Complete Blood Count (CBC)

Epstein-Barr Virus (EBV) Antibody Tests

See Infectious Mononucleosis Tests

Erythrocyte Sedimentation Rate (ESR)

See Sedimentation Rate

Esophagogastro-duodenoscopy (EGD) Endoscopy, Gastroscopy

Endoscopic Imaging

This examination allows the physician to visualize the esophagus, stomach, and duodenum through a fiberoptic scope.

Indications
- Evaluate ulcers, epigastric or substernal pain, upper GI diseases or injuries, anatomical variations, dyspepsia.
- Diagnose and control bleeding and remove foreign bodies, obtain biopsies and specimens for laboratory studies.

Expected Test Outcomes
Esophagus, stomach, and upper duodenum normal in appearance (esophagus = yellow-pink; stomach = orange-red; duodenal bulk = red).

Test Outcome Deviations
- Abnormal findings reveal upper GI bleeding/hemorrhage sites, diverticula; neoplasms, both benign and malignant, varices; esophageal rings, stenoses, ulcers; inflammatory processes, and hiatal hernia.

Interfering Factors

- Chemical ingestion or history of alcohol abuse.

Procedure

- A topical anesthetic is applied to patient's throat and patient is placed in a left lateral position with knees flexed. Intravenous sedation is administered. If teeth are intact, a mouthpiece is inserted. The endoscope is gently passed through the opening in the mouthpiece into esophagus, stomach, and duodenum. Air passed through scope distends the area being examined so that better visualization is achieved. Biopsies and brushings for cytology are taken; photos provide a permanent record of the visual exam. As the scope is withdrawn, it also draws out some of the air.

Nursing Role

Use nursing process model following pre-, intra-, and posttest care guidelines in Chapter 1. See page 8 for list of appropriate nursing diagnoses.

Nursing Diagnosis

- Knowledge deficit related to lack or misinterpretation of information provided about purpose and EGD procedure.
- Anxiety related to need for participation in EGD.
- Powerlessness related to lack of control over hospital environment.
- High risk for aspiration related to manipulation of Gl tract.

....
CLINICAL ALERT

◊ Obtain signed, witnessed consent for EGD.
....

Pretest Care

- Explain procedure, purpose of exam, and need for sedation and local anesthetic. Check for allergies to drugs. Fasting state for at least 6 hours pretest. Remove dentures, jewelry, hairpieces, glasses, tight clothing. Explain that a full feeling or pressure may be felt with movement of the scope and introduction of air. Have patient void if necessary.
- Administer prescribed medications and record baseline vital signs.

Intratest Care

- Assist with positioning patient's head during the exam. Monitor vital signs as necessary; be alert to adverse medication reactions. Send properly prepared specimens to laboratory. See Appendix B for standards regarding IV conscious sedation.
- A CLO test (campylobacter-like organism) may be done if *Helicobacter pylori* is suspected as causative agent for active chronic gastritis, duodenal or gastric ulcers, or nonulcer dyspepsia. Gastric mucosal biopsies are taken and immersed into test gel for rapid urea organisms. Readings are taken at 20-minute, 1-hour, and 3-hour intervals. An orange gel, after 30 minutes, is usually positive for *H. pylori*. The gel will turn a magenta color after several hours. If gel remains yellow, test is negative. Document results.
- A videoendoscopic evaluation of dysphagia (VEED) test may be done as part of the EGD. Pudding and crackers are swallowed and then tracked on video. Views of the nasopharynx, laryngopharynx, and larynx assist in evaluating aspiration associated with dysphagia.

Posttest Care

- Allow nothing by mouth until swallowing reflex returns (usually about 2 hours). Take and record vital signs according to protocols or patient status. Keep in side-lying position if patient remains sedated. Provide saline gargle for a sore throat after swallowing reflex is intact.

••••••••••••••
CLINICAL ALERT

◊ Signs of perforation include pain with swallowing and neck motion, substernal or epigastric pain, shoulder pain, and dyspnea, or abdominal pain, back pain, cyanosis, fever, and pleural effusion.

••••••••••••••

Estrogen Total,   *Urine and Blood*
Estrogen Fractions/
Estradiol (E₂) Estriol (E₃)

These tests are used along with gonadotropins to measure hormone levels.

Indications

- Evaluate estradiol for menstrual and fertility problems in women and feminization in men.
- Investigate estriol for estrogen producing tumors; monitor pregnancy and fetal well-being.

Expected Test Outcomes

Vary widely between women and men, pregnancy, menopausal state, and follicular, ovulatory, and luteal stage of menstrual cycle.

Total Estrogen—Urine

Male: 4–25 µg/24 h
Female
   Nonpregnant: 4–60 µg/24 h
   Pregnant 1st trimester: 0–800 µg/24 h
   Pregnant 2nd trimester: 800–5,000 µg/24 h
   Pregnant 3rd trimester: 5,000–50,000 µg/24 h
   Child: < 12 y old: 1 µg/24 h
   Post-puberty: same as adult above

Estriol—Urine

Male: 1–11 µg/24 h
Female
   Follicular phase: 0–14 µg/24 h
   Ovulatory phase: 13–54 µg/24 h
   Luteal phase: 8–60 µg/24 h
   Postmenopausal: 0–11 µg/24 h
   Pregnant 1st trimester: 0–800 µg/24 h
   Pregnant 2nd trimester: 800–12,000 µg/24 h
   Pregnant 3rd trimester: 5,000–50,000 µg/24 h

Estradiol—Serum

Child: 1–6 y—3–10 pg/mL; 8–12 y—< 30 pg/mL.

OVULATING FEMALES	DAY	LH PEAK (PG/ML)
follicular phase	–12	10–50
midcycle	–4	60–200
luteal phase	+2	50–155
	+6	60–260
	+12	15–115

Estriol—Serum

Gestational Age (wk)	ng/mL
34	5.3–18.3
35	5.2–26.4
36	8.2–28.1
37	8.0–30.1
38	8.6–38.0
39	7.2–34.3
40	9.6–28.9

Test Outcome Deviations

- *Increased estrogen* levels associated with ovarian tumors, some testicular tumors, tumors or hyperplasia of the adrenal cortex, precocious puberty, corpus luteum cyst, liver disease, and pregnancy.
- *Decreased estrogen* levels associated with hypofunction or dysfunction of pituitary and adrenal glands, primary ovarian malfunction, menopause, anovulatory bleeding, inadequate luteal phase, anorexia nervosa, psychogenic stress.
- *Decreased estriol* levels associated with placental insufficiency, fetal distress—an abrupt drop of 40% or more on two consecutive days—fetal outcome is considered favorable if the movement is upward; malnutrition, and renal disease.

Interfering Factors

- Drugs which can cause false negatives include vitamins, some phenothiazines; tetracycline can cause false positives.

Procedure

- Serum (10 mL) obtained.
- A 24-hour urine sample can be collected using a preservative and refrigeration. See specimen collection guidelines in Chapter 2. General information for 24-hour urine collection is in Appendix E.

Nursing Role

Use nursing process model following pre-, intra-, and posttest care guidelines in Chapter 1. See page 8 for list of appropriate nursing diagnoses.

Nursing Diagnosis

- Knowledge deficit related to lack of or misinterpretation of information provided about purpose and procedure.

- Anxiety and fear related to nature of test, test outcome, and possible need for further treatment.
- Potential for noncompliance to test protocols related to presence of high anxiety, confusion, denial.

Pretest Care

- Assess patient compliance, patient knowledge base prior to explaining test purpose and procedure, and anxiety about testing of sex hormones.

Intratest Care

- No restriction of food or fluids required. Accurate test results depend upon proper collection, preservation, and labeling. Be sure to include test start and completion times. Note on laboratory requisition the phase of patient's menstrual cycle and if taking any sex-related hormones.

Posttest Care

- Evaluate patient outcome; provide counseling and support as appropriate.

Ethanol

See Alcohol

Fasting Blood Sugar

See Blood Glucose Tests

Ferritin

See Iron Tests

Folic Acid (Folate) and Vitamin B_{12} (VB_{12})   Blood

These B vitamin measurements are usually tested in conjunction with one another to diagnose macrocytic anemia.

Indications

- Differential diagnosis of anemia.
- Diagnose pernicious anemia and leukemia.

Expected Test Outcomes

- *Folic acid*: 2–20 µg/L.
- *Vitamin B$_{12}$*: Women 20–79 y—190–765 ng/L; Males 0–29 y—281–1079 ng/L; and 70–79 y—152–630 ng/L.
- Vitamin B$_{12}$ (unsaturated binding capacity): 1000–2000 pg/mL

Test Outcome Deviations

- *Vitamin B$_{12}$ decreases* in pernicious anemia, malabsorption and inflammatory bowel disease; gastrostomy/gastric resection, Zollinger-Ellison syndrome, hemodialysis, and multiple myeloma.
- *Vitamin B$_{12}$ increases* in chronic granulocytic leukemia, myelomonocytic leukemia, liver disease, some cancers and uremia.
- *Unsaturated binding capacity increases* in polycythemia and chronic myelocytic leukemia.
- *Unsaturated binding capacity decreases* in hepatic cirrhosis and hepatitis.
- *Folic acid decreases* in macrocytic and megaloblastic anemia, insufficient dietary intake, alcoholism, liver disease, hemolytic disorders, malignancies, and hemodialysis.

Interfering Factors

- Altered outcomes in persons with recent diagnostic or therapeutic doses of radionuclides, high vitamin C doses, oral contraceptives, aspirin, and vegetarian diet.
- Pregnancy, smoking, and age affect outcome.

Procedure

- Vitamin B$_{12}$: a fasting serum sample of 7–10 mL is obtained before, injection of vitamin B$_{12}$ following collection guidelines in Chapter 2.
- Folic acid: whole blood sample 5–7 mL is obtained.

Nursing Role

Use nursing process model following pre-, intra-, and posttest care guidelines in Chapter 1. See page 8 for list of appropriate nursing diagnoses.

Nursing Diagnosis

- Knowledge deficit related to lack or misinterpretation of information provided about purpose and procedure.
- High risk for infection, bleeding, or hematoma following venipuncture.

Pretest Care

- Explain purpose and procedures. No food overnight. Water is permitted.

Posttest Care

- Evaluate patient outcomes and counsel and monitor appropriately regarding test outcome deviations. Advise regarding foods high in vitamin B_{12} and folic acid.

Follicle-Stimulating Hormone (FSH); Luteinizing Hormone (LH)
Timed Urine

This test measures gonadotropic hormones FSH and LH to determine whether a gonadal insufficiency is primary or due to insufficient stimulation by the pituitary hormones.

Indications

- Evaluate primary ovarian or testicular failure.
- Measure urine FSH and LH in children with endocrine problems related to precocious puberty.
- Monitor ovulatory cycles of in vitro fertilization patients.

Expected Test Outcomes

	FSH	LH
Men	1–20 IU/24 h	5–20 IU/24 h
Women	5–20 IU/24 h	5–15 IU/24 h follicular phase
Post-menopausal	30–440 IU/24 h	50–100 IU/24 h
Midcycle peak	15–30 IU/24 h	30–95 IU/24 h
Child (prepubertal)	<10 IU/24 h	

Test Outcome Deviations

- *Decreased FSH* levels occur in feminizing and masculinizing ovarian tumors where production is inhibited as a result of increased estrogen, failure of pituitary or hypothalamus, anorexia nervosa, neoplasm of testes or adrenal glands that secrete estrogens or androgens, and precocious puberty related to adrenal tumors.
- *Increased FSH* levels occur in Turner's syndrome, hypogonadism (primary), complete testicular feminization syndrome, precocious puberty (idiopathic), Klinefelter's syndrome, and menopause.

- *Both FSH and LH increased* in primary gonadal failure, complete testicular feminization syndrome, and precocious puberty.
- *Decreased FSH and LH* in failure of pituitary or hypothalamus.

Interfering Factors

- Certain drugs can cause false negatives in FSH levels such as testosterone, estrogens, and oral contraceptives.

Procedure

- Urine is collected for 24 hours either with a preservative or refrigerated only. See timed specimen collection and handling guidelines in Chapter 2 and Appendix E. Check with your laboratory about policy.
- Note drugs patient is taking on lab slip or computer screen.

Nursing Role

Use nursing process model following pre-, intra-, and posttest care guidelines in Chapter 1. See page 8 for list of appropriate nursing diagnoses.

Nursing Diagnosis

- Knowledge deficit related to lack or misinterpretation of information provided about purpose, procedure, and need for patient cooperation.
- Anxiety and fear related to test outcome and possible need for further treatment.
- Noncompliance related to inability to follow specimen collection protocols.

Pretest Care

- Assess patient compliance and patient knowledge base prior to explaining test purpose and procedure.

Intratest Care

- Accurate test results depend on proper collection, preservation, and labeling. Be sure to include test start and completion times.

Posttest Care

- Evaluate patient outcome. Provide counseling and support as appropriate.

Free Thyroxine Index (FTI)

See Thyroid Function Tests

Fungal Antibody Tests **Blood** (Histoplasmosis, Blastomycosis, Coccidioidomycosis Cryptococcal Infection)

These tests are done to diagnose fungal infections involving the deep tissues and internal organs caused by *Histoplasma capsulatum*, *Blastomyces*, *Coccidioides immitis*, and *Cryptococcus*.

Indications

- Evaluate fungus infection involving respiratory tract in persons with signs and symptoms and possible history of inhalation of spores from sources such as contaminated dusts, soil, and bird droppings.
- Assess patients who have symptoms of pulmonary or meningeal infection.
- Evaluate cryptococcus infection in patients with predisposing conditions such as lymphoma, sarcoidosis, steroid therapy, or AIDS.

Procedure

- Serum (7 mL) is obtained by venipuncture following collection guidelines in Chapter 2.
- Antibodies to fungi are detected by either complement-fixation or immunodiffusion tests.

Expected Test Outcomes

- Complement-fixation (CF) titer: <1:8.
- Immunodiffusion: negative for antibodies or antigens to these fungi.
- Cryptococcus antibodies or antigens: 1:4 titer is suggestive of cryptococcal infection; 1:8 or greater titer indicates active infection. Antigen titer is usually proportional to extent of infection. Failure of titer to fall during therapy suggests inadequate therapy.

Test Outcome Deviations

- Antibodies to coccidioidomycosis, blastomycosis, and histoplasmosis appear early in the disease (from first to fourth weeks) and then disappear.

Interfering Factors

- Antibodies against fungi may be found in blood of apparently normal people who live in an area where the fungus is endemic.

- In tests for blastomycosis, there may be cross-reactions with histoplasmosis.
- False positives for cryptococcus are seen in patients with elevated rheumatoid factor levels.

Nursing Role

Use nursing process model following pre-, intra-, and posttest care guidelines in Chapter 1. See page 8 for list of appropriate nursing diagnoses.

Nursing Diagnosis

- Knowledge deficit related to lack of information or possible misinterpretation of information provided about purpose and procedure.
- High risk of injury or infection related to venipuncture.

Pretest Care

- Assess patient's knowledge of test and travel history to endemic areas. Explain purpose and blood test procedure. No fasting is required.

Posttest Care

- Evaluate patient outcomes and counsel appropriately. Advise patient that additional procedures such as skin tests, cultures, and lumbar puncture for CS fluid may be required to identify particular fungus involved.

Gallbladder and Biliary Scan, GB Scan, Hepatobiliary Scan

Nuclear Medicine Scan Imaging

This nuclear study is done to visualize the gallbladder and determine patency of the biliary system.

Indications

- Investigate persons with abdominal pain.
- Evaluate cholecystitis and differentiate obstructive from nonobstructive jaundice.
- Evaluate biliary atresia and postsurgery biliary assessment.

Expected Test Outcomes

- Normal gallbladder, biliary system, and duodenum.

Test Outcome Deviations

- Acute and chronic cholecystitis, gallstones, biliary atresia, strictures, and lesions.

Interfering Factors

- Elevated bilirubin (>10 mg/dL) and some pain medications may affect reliable outcomes.
- Total parenteral nutrition (TPN) and long-term fast.

Procedure

- Radionuclide technetium is injected intravenously. A series of images begins immediately and at 10–15 minute intervals for 60–90 minutes. In the event of biliary obstruction, delayed scans may be obtained at 4–24 hours.
- In some patients, choleocystokinine (CCK) is administered to differentiate acute from chronic cholecystitis.

Nursing Role

Use nursing process model following pre-, intra-, and posttest care guidelines in Chapter 1. See page 8 for list of appropriate nursing diagnoses.

Nursing Diagnosis

- Knowledge deficit related to lack of or misinterpretation of information provided about purpose, procedure, and radionuclide administration.
- High risk for injury related to radiation hazard of nuclear scan.

Pretest Care

- Explain purpose and procedure. Record accurate weight. Fast at least 2 hours. A 24-hour or longer fast is to be avoided. Reassure regarding safety of injection of radiopharmaceutical. See alphabetical list for nuclear scans overview.
- Give no opiates or morphine-based pain medication 2–6 hours prior to test due to treatment interference of the radiopharmaceutical.
- See Nuclear Medicine Scans: Overview.

Intratest Care

• Provide reassurance and support.

Posttest Care

• Evaluate patient outcomes and counsel appropriately.
• Assess IV site for signs of infection.
• Dispose of body fluids and excretions following routine procedures unless patient is also receiving therapeutic doses of
  radiopharmaceuticals.
• Pregnant staff and visitors are to avoid prolonged contact for
  24–48 hours following radioactive administration.

Gallbladder and Biliary System Ultrasound, GB Sonogram, Echogram

Ultrasound Imaging

This noninvasive procedure is used to visualize and diagnose
gallbladder, surrounding liver tissue, and bile duct diseases
and is the procedure of choice when a gallbladder x-ray is contraindicated.

Indications

• Initial study for persons with chronic upper right quadrant
  pain.
• Differentiate gallbladder from heart disease, detect gallstones
  or chronic cholecystitis and evaluate nonfunctioning gallbladder that does not visualize on x-ray.
• Guide fine needle aspiration for biopsy.

Expected Test Outcomes

Normal gallbladder size and position of gallbladder and bile
ducts. Normal liver tissue.

Test Outcome Deviations

• Presence of inflammation, cancer and polyps of gallbladder,
  gallstones in gallbladder and bile ducts; dilatations, strictures, and obstructions of biliary tree.

Interfering Factors

• Barium from previous procedures, presence of gas, and obesity affect test outcomes.

Procedure

- Position patient on back (usually supine, sidelying, or upright position) on examining table. A conductive gel is applied to skin over area to be examined.
- A hand-held ultrasound transducer is slowly moved over specific area of body. Patient is instructed to control breathing pattern while imaging pictures are taken. Time-frame is approximately 20–30 minutes depending upon other procedures or diagnostic modalities needed.

Nursing Role

Use nursing process model following pre-, intra-, and posttest care guidelines in Chapter 1. See page 8 for list of appropriate nursing diagnoses.

Nursing Diagnosis

- Knowledge deficit related to lack or possible misinterpretation of information provided about procedure, purpose, and preparation.
- Decisional conflict related to test outcome, the need for gallbladder surgery versus medical treatment, and corresponding life-styles changes.

Pretest Care

- Explain purpose and ultrasound procedure—no radiation is involved. Tell patient the test is painless. Emphasize pretest food and drink restrictions. No food 6–12 hours prior to test; water is usually permitted.
- Administer enemas if ordered pretest.

Intratest Care

- On occasion, a fatty substance will be given orally to assess contractility of gallbladder.

Posttest Care

- Remove gel or instruct patient to cleanse abdomen of remaining gel.
- Evaluate patient outcomes, provide support and counseling.

••••••••••••••
CLINICAL ALERT

◊ Scans cannot be effectively performed over open wounds or dressings.

◊ This exam must be performed before barium or more than 24 hours after barium administration.

◊ Nonfasting will result in inadequate visualization of gallbladder.

◊ Patient must agree to and sign a surgical permit prior to performance of an ultrasound guided biopsy or other interventional procedures.

·············

Gallbladder X-Ray— GB X-Ray, Gallbladder Radiography, Cholecystography, Oral Cholecystogram, Gallbladder Series

X-Ray Imaging with Contrast

This x-ray study uses an oral iodine contrast substance to visualize the functioning of the gallbladder and diagnose gallbladder disease or gallstones.

Indications

• Use in conjunction with gallbladder ultrasound to verify calculi, evaluate suspected cholelithiasis, and identify congenital gallbladder abnormalities.

Expected Test Outcomes

Normal structure and functioning (filling, concentration, contraction, and emptying) of gallbladder and ducts. No stones.

Test Outcome Deviations

• Presence of cholecystitis, cholelithiasis, polyps, tumors, and cystic duct obstruction, congenital malformation, presence of gas and no visualization of a gallbladder (only occurs in chronically inflamed or many stones).

Interfering Factors

• Poor intestinal absorption, barium remaining in GI tract from previous procedures, obstructed bile duct (will affect absorption and expected test outcome), and noncompliance with test preparation procedure.

• Test is effective only when liver function is normal and liver is capable of excreting iodine contrast into the bile.

Procedure

- A series of x-rays of upper right quadrant are made with patient assuming these positions: lying on abdomen, lying with right side elevated away from table, sitting, or standing.
- A high-fat substance may be given orally or intravenously to cause gallbladder to contract and empty. X-rays follow 20–60 minutes after this.

Nursing Role

Use nursing process model following pre-, intra-, and posttest care guidelines in Chapter 1. See page 8 for list of appropriate nursing diagnoses.

Nursing Diagnosis

- Knowledge deficit related to lack or possible misinterpretation of information provided about procedure, purpose, and preparation.
- High risk of injury related to allergic reaction to iodine contrast media.
- Decisional conflict related to test outcome and need for gallbladder surgery versus medical treatment and corresponding life-style changes.
- Potential noncompliance related to specifics of test preparation.

Pretest Care

- Assess for contraindications for testing such as jaundice, vomiting and diarrhea, allergy to iodine, pregnancy, other abdominal inflammatory processes, and bilirubin elevated greater than 3 mg/dL. Explain purpose and x-ray procedure and special test requirements.
- See Appendix A for standards regarding contrast media precautions.

....
CLINICAL ALERT

◊ Consider the following when scheduling gallbladder series tests: (1) thyroid testing, scans, and blood work done prior to GB x-rays; (2) barium studies performed after GB studies; and (3) upper GI series may be done at same time as GB series.

◊ Special test requirements include: eat fat-restricted meal evening before test; take each iodine med with a full glass of water unless on a fluid restriction diet; stool softener or enema may be ordered. No food permitted after administration of iodine capsules until test is completed.
....

Intratest Care

- Be sure patient gets to x-ray department in a timely way so that all x-rays in GB studies are completed accurately.

Posttest Care

- Provide fluids, food, and rest after examination is completed. Observe patient for allergic reaction to iodine contrast substance. See Appendix A for specific standards. If diarrhea occurs, provide additional oral fluids at once.
- Repeat testing may be necessary if gallbladder does not visualize.

___

Gamma Glutamyl Transferase (GGT); Gamma Glutamyl Transpeptidase (GGT); Gamma Glutamyl Transferase (GGT)

See Liver Function Tests

___

Gastric Analysis (Tube Gastric Analysis)

Gastric Fluid

This test is done to examine the contents of the stomach for the presence of abnormal substances such as blood, bacteria, and drugs and to measure gastric acidity.

Indications

- Diagnose gastric or duodenal ulcers, pyloric or intestinal obstruction, and Zollinger-Ellison syndrome, pernicious anemia, and carcinoma of the stomach.
- Determine cause of Gl bleeding, effectiveness of medical or surgical antiulcer therapy.
- Cytologic exam for culture of gastric washings to identify mycobacterial infection when previous sputum tests were negative.

Expected Test Outcomes

- 5 mL of clear or opalescent fluid; no food, no blood, drugs, or bile present.
- Cytologic culture negative for mycobacterial organisms.
- Fasting, basal acid output (BAO)—without stimulation: 2–5 mEq/h.

- Maximal acid output (MAO) or normal secretory ability using a gastric stimulant such as histamine: 10–20 mEq/h. Elderly patients frequently have lower levels of gastric hydrochloric acid.

Test Outcome Deviations

- *Decreased levels* of gastric acid (hypochlorhydria) in pernicious anemia, gastric malignancy, atrophic gastritis, adrenal insufficiency, vertiligo, rheumatoid arthritis, thyroid toxicosis, chronic renal failure, and postvagotomy.
- *Increased levels* of gastric acid (hypersecretion and hyperchlorhydria) in peptic ulcer (duodenal), Zollinger-Ellison syndrome, hyperplasia and hyperfunction of antral gastric cells, and following massive small intestine resection.

Interfering Factors

- Presence of barium left in stomach from previous x-ray studies and lubricant used to insert nasogastric tubes can distort cells.
- Medications such as antacids, anticholinergics, histamine blockers (ie, Tagamet; food, fluid, and smoking alter gastric acid secretion.
- Diabetics that require insulin treatment and surgical vagotomy alter test results.
- Problems related to passing nasogastric tube, such as previous nasal surgery, trauma, or deviated septum.

Procedure

- Gastric analysis specimens are collected in a fasting state, following endoscopy or insertion of a nasogastric (NG) tube. NG tubes may be inserted by properly trained nurses, using specific protocols from agencies' policy and procedure manuals. If both basal and stimulation gastric analysis are done, procedures usually take 2 1/2–3 hours. See Intratest Care.

Nursing Role

Use nursing process model following pre-, intra-, and posttest care guidelines in Chapter 1. See page 8 for list of appropriate nursing diagnoses.

Nursing Diagnosis

- Knowledge deficit related to lack of information or possible misinterpretation of information about procedure, equipment, purpose, and preparation.

- Potential for altered comfort related to the insertion of NG tube and numerous collection of specimens.
- Potential for noncompliance related to inadequate test preparation (ie, did not fast, continued to smoke or take medication that interferes with test).
- High risk of injury related to passing of nasogastric tube.

Pretest Care

- Assess for contraindications for procedure such as: patients with carcinoid syndrome, congestive heart failure, or hypertension—histamine for test may exacerbate conditions.
- Record baseline vital signs and remove loose dentures prior to test.
- Explain purpose of test and actual procedure. Inform patient that there may be some discomfort when the nasogastric tube is inserted. Instruct to restrict food, fluids and smoking 8–12 hours prior to test (usually NPO after midnight). Restrict anticholinergics, cholinergics, adrenergic blockers, antacids, steroids, alcohol, and coffee for at least 24 hours before test.

Intratest Care

- Devise a method of communication for patient prior to insertion of nasogastric tube, for example, raise index finger to indicate "wait" before proceeding. Explain that panting, mouth-breathing, and swallowing will facilitate tube insertion. Observe for signs of distress such as coughing or cyanosis when inserting tube. Initial gastric acid is aspirated and discarded, usually with a syringe. Four subsequent specimens are then collected at 15-minute intervals. These are labeled BAO with patient's name, time, and specimen number. A gastric stimulant is then administered—betazole hydrochloride (Histalez), or histamine phosphate IM; or pentagastrin subcutaneously.

• • • • • • • • • • • • • •
CLINICAL ALERT

◊ If histamine is injected, inform patient that flushing, dizziness, headache, faintness, and numbness of extremities and abdomen may occur during or immediately after testing. Advise patient to report changes immediately. Have epinephrine ready to treat for shock, if histamine is injected.
• • • • • • • • • • • • • •

- Specimens are collected via low suction over a period of 1–2 hours at 15-minute intervals (depending upon medication given). Label specimen as to patient's name, date, time, and MAO specimen. Remove tube after all specimens are collected. Document date and time of procedure, type and size of tube used, specimen collected, physician's name, specific procedure, color, consistency and amount of gastric fluid obtained, patient's response, ability to comply with test until completion, complications, interventions, and, finally, disposition of the specimen.

••••••••••••
CLINICAL ALERT
◊ Specimens for acid fast bacillus (AFB) culture need to be warm when taken to lab and personnel should be alerted to nature of specimen as soon as possible.
••••••••••••

Posttest Care
• Monitor vital signs and observe for possible side effects of stimulants. Observe for respiratory bleeding or distress and gastrointestinal bleeding (may be sign of perforation). Provide nasal/oral care after tube removal. Allow patient to rest as test may exhaust some patients. Provide food or fluids as tolerated/or ordered. If any local anesthetic was used, wait until gag and swallow reflexes have adequately returned.

• Counsel patient in relation to posttest deviations and the need to alter lifestyle, such as stop smoking, alcohol, diet changes (caffeine or stimulants), stress reduction, and medication or surgical interventions.

━━━━━

Gastric X-Ray Radiography, Upper GI Study, Esophagus and Stomach X-Ray, Small Bowel Study

X-Ray Imaging with Contrast

These exams use both fluoroscopic and x-ray techniques to visualize the upper gastrointestinal tract and provide views of the distal esophagus, stomach, duodenum, and first part of the jejunum. The small bowel study is generally ordered as a continuation of the upper gastrointestinal (UGI) to follow and document the filling of the entire small bowel.

Indications

- Rule out ulcers, obstructions, and hernias.
- Evaluate gastric pain and swallowing difficulties.
- Detect presence of Crohn's disease.

Expected Test Outcomes

Normal size, contour, motility, and peristaltic patterns of the esophagus, stomach, and duodenum. Normal small intestine position, contour, and filling.

Test Outcome Deviations

- Congenital abnormalities, ulcers, masses, foreign bodies, polyps, diverticula, gastritis and reflux, hiatal hernia, and Crohn's disease.

Interfering Factors

- Retention of food or fluid residue will obscure complete visualization of GI structures.
- Optimal GI studies depend upon patient's ability to consume contrast media orally. Inability to do so will compromise exam quality.
- Severe obesity adversely affects image quality.

Procedure

- After NPO for approximately 8 hours prior to exam, an oral contrast agent, usually barium, is administered orally to outline the GI contents. Follow-up x-rays are performed after fluoroscopic exam. Exam time is 20–45 minutes.
- For small bowel study, the procedure is as above, but exam time much longer. Since peristaltic pattern, general activity, and presence of disease influences how quickly contrast moves through the intestinal tract, this study can vary from minutes to several hours.

Nursing Role

Use nursing process model following pre-, intra-, and posttest care guidelines in Chapter 1. See page 8 for list of appropriate nursing diagnoses.

Nursing Diagnosis

- Knowledge deficit related to lack or possible misinterpretation of information provided about procedure and purpose.

- Anxiety and fear related to unfamiliarity with diagnostic procedure and equipment.
- Ineffective coping related to test outcome and inability to accept diagnosis of disease.
- High risk of injury related to administration of barium contrast.

Pretest Care

- Assess for test contraindications (pregnancy).
- Explain exam purpose and procedure. Assure patient that test is painless. No food or beverage is allowed for approximately 8 hours prior to study. Make certain that jewelry and metallic objects are removed from abdominal area. See Appendix A for standards regarding contrast media precautions.

Intratest Care

- Encourage patient to follow breathing and positional instructions.

Posttest Care

- Provide fluids, food, and rest after study. Administer laxatives if ordered.
- Observe and record stool color/consistency to determine if all barium has been eliminated from bowel.
- Evaluate patient outcomes; provide support and counseling.

Globulins

See Protein

Glucose; Fasting Blood Sugar (FBS)

See Blood Glucose Tests

Glucose Tolerance Test, Oral (OGTT)

See Blood Glucose/Sugar Tests

Glycosylated Hemoglobin (HbA$_{1c}$); Glycohemoglobin (G-Hb)

See Blood Glucose Monitoring

Gynecologic Sonogram— Pelvic Ultrasound Pelvic Mass Diagnosis

Ultrasound Imaging

This noninvasive study is used to visualize the soft tissue structures located in the pelvic cavity including the urinary bladder, uterus, ovaries, and major pelvic blood vessels.

Indications

- Determine size and characteristics of a palpable pelvic mass and location of intrauterine contraceptive device.
- Assess structural deviations which may cause menstrual irregularities and cause infertility.
- Rule out ectopic pregnancy.
- Monitor follicular development in patients undergoing ovulation induction.

Expected Test Outcomes

Normal sonographic image of urinary bladder, vagina, uterus, ovaries, and adnexal structures.

Test Outcome Deviations

- Simple and benign physiologic cysts, fibroids, pelvic inflammatory disease, endometriosis, solid ovarian lesions, growth or spread of a tumor.
- Inward distortion of bladder wall is suggestive of pressure from an external mass; thickened or irregular bladder walls are often associated with bladder masses.

Interfering Factors

- Gas or barium in bowel overlying pelvic contents will obscure image. Results may be compromised if patient is obese or has a retroverted uterus. Success of transabdominal scans is dependent upon maintenance of a full bladder during study.

Procedure

Transabdominal approach requires a fully distended urinary bladder.

- A coupling medium, generally gel, is applied to area under study in order to promote transmission of sound. A handheld transducer is slowly moved across skin during imaging procedure. Exam time is about 30 minutes.

Transvaginal (endovaginal) approach does not require a full bladder.

- A small vaginal transducer, sheathed and lubricated, is inserted into vagina to a depth no greater than 8 cm. Scans are performed using slight rotational movements of transducer handle. Exam time is about 15–30 minutes.

Nursing Role

Use nursing process model following pre-, intra-, and posttest care guidelines in Chapter 1. See page 8 for list of appropriate nursing diagnoses.

Nursing Diagnosis

- Knowledge deficit related to lack or possible misinterpretation of information provided about procedure, purpose, and preparation.
- Ineffective coping related to test outcome and inability to accept diagnosis of bladder, vagina, uterus, and ovarian disorders.

Pretest Care

- Explain exam purpose and procedure. No radiation is used and test is painless. Test preparation, in most cases, requires a full bladder which will require 32 ounces of water or clear fluid consumed 1–2 hours before procedure. Instruct patient not to void until exam is completed. Discomfort associated with a very full bladder is expected.
- Under certain conditions, a transvaginal approach is used which does not require bladder filling.

· · · · · · · · · · · · · ·
CLINICAL ALERT

◊ If patient is NPO or in certain emergency situations, patient may be catheterized and bladder filled via catheter.
◊ Patient must agree to and sign a surgical permit prior to any ultrasound-guided interventional technique such as oocyte retrieval.

· · · · · · · · · · · · · ·

Intratest Care

- Encourage patient if maintaining a distended bladder is difficult.

Posttest Care

- Remove or instruct patient to remove any residual gel from skin.
- Instruct patient to empty bladder frequently upon completion of full-bladder study.
- Evaluate patient outcomes; provide support and counseling as necessary.

Heart Scans

Nuclear Medicine Scan Imaging

Cardiac Imaging, Myocardial Perfusion, PYP, Thallium Stress, Gated Scan, MUGA, First Pass, Nitro Test, Heart Shunt

These nuclear studies involve the intravenous injection of a radiopharmaceutical to measure heart chamber dimensions and function, and investigate myocardial infarction, coronary artery disease, and chest pain.

Indications

Pyrophospate (PYP) Heart Scan

- Diagnose acute myocardial infarction and differentiate between new and old infarcts.
- Use when ECG and enzyme studies are not definitive and commonly performed before and after open heart surgery.

Myocardial Perfusion Stress Imaging

- Rule out myocardial ischemia, differentiate between ischemia and infarct, and quantitate the degree and location of ischemia.

Dipyridamole/Persantine Imaging

- Use in person unable to exercise to achieve desired stress; for patients with lung disease, amputation, spinal cord injury, multiple sclerosis, morbid obesity, and taking beta blockers.

Gated Equilibrium Heart Scan

- Evaluate regional wall motion primarily on left ventricle and determine quantitative data (eg, ejection fraction on left ventricular function).

Nitro Test

- Evaluate effects of nitroglycerine on heart performance.

First Pass (When a Bolus of ^{99m}Tc First Passes Through the Right Heart, Lungs and Left Heart)

- Evaluate both right and left ventricular function and alternate to mutigated acquisition (MUGA) to obtain ejection fractions and quantitative data.

Heart Shunt (Heart Chamber Study)

- Determine left-to-right and right-to-left cardiac shunts and assess conventional cardiac defects in children.

Expected Test Outcomes

PYP Heart Scan

- No myocardial uptake.

Myocardial Perfusion Stress and Dipyridamole/ Persantine Imaging

- Normal myocardial uptake; no areas of ischemia; normal stress test: electrocardiogram (ECG) and blood pressure normal.

Gated Equilibrium Heart Scan

- Normal wall motion, ejection fractions, and velocity.

Nitro Test

- Normal nitro test: blood pressure within expected limits.

First Pass

- Blood flow is equal throughout the myocardium.
- Normal ejection fraction.

Cardiac Shunt

- Normal shunt scan: pulmonary transit times and normal sequence or chamber filling.

Test Outcome Deviations

- Location and extent of myocardial infarction; abnormal cardiac output; perfusion defects associated with ischemic heart disease, cardiac hypertrophy; abnormal MUGA status associated with congestive heart failure; poor ventricular function.
- Abnormal heart shunts and ejection fractions.

Interfering Factors

- Long-acting nitrates. Discontinue 8–12 hours prior to test.

- False positive for infarct PYP scans in presence of chest wall trauma, recent cardioversion, and unstable angina.
- Gated and PYP stress studies interfere with other nuclear tests if they are done on same day.

Procedures

PYP Heart Scan Procedure

- This myocardial scan involves a 3–6 hour waiting period for the patient after intravenous injection of the radionuclide. During this waiting period, radioactive material will accumulate in heart muscle.
- Imaging period takes 15–30 minutes, during which time the patient must lie quietly on an examining table.

Myocardial Perfusion Stress Imaging Procedure

- Before the stress test is begun, an intravenous line is started, and ECG leads and blood pressure cuff are attached.
- With thallium 201, the procedure is as follows: When cardiologist has determined that patient has reached maximum heart stress using treadmill (10–30 minutes), an injection of radioactive thallium is given. Patient then lies down on the scanning table and scanning is begun immediately. Imaging period is about a half hour. A repeat scan is done approximately 4 hours later at rest to check redistribution.
- With ^{99m}Tc Sestamibi, the procedure has several options: (a) same-day rest followed by stress 3–4 hours later; (b) same-day stress followed by rest 3–4 hours later; (c) 2-day sequence with rest on first day followed by stress 24 hours later; (d) 2-day sequence with stress on first day followed by rest 24 hours later. With any option for ^{99m}Tc Sestamibi, scanning begins approximately 1 hour after radioactive injection for both stress and rest.

Dipyridamole/Persantine Imaging Procedure

- Either of these drugs are administered in place of physical stress. Dipyridamole may be administered orally as an option.
- Blood pressure, heart rate, and ECG are monitored for any changes during persantine infusion. Aminophylline will be given if vital signs change radically.

Gated Equilibrium Heart Scan Procedure

- This scan may be performed with or without stress testing and is usually performed in conjunction with heart wall motion study. The test could be performed at bedside if necessary. The patient's own red blood cells become labeled with ^{99m}Tc stannous pyrophosphate.

Nitroglycerine Test

- A resting MUGA is done for a baseline study. Nitroglycerine is given, another scan is taken, nitroglycerine is given again, and scans are taken until the level of blood pressure desired by the cardiologist is reached. Total study time is approximately 1.5 hours.

First Pass Test Procedure

- An intravenous line is established in the basilic (medial) vein of forearm. A 3-way stopcock is attached with the radioactive med in one port and a 10-cc saline flush in the other.
- The injection uses a rapid bolus technique followed by the saline flush with the patient under the camera.
- In many situations, the patient is monitored by ECG.
- The actual scan time is less than 2 minutes.

Cardiac Shunt Procedure

- A radionuclide is injected in the external jugular vein to ensure a compact bolus with patient lying on the back with head slightly raised. Total patient time is approximately 30 minutes; actual scan time 5 minutes. A resting MUGA is performed with *each* shunt study.

Nursing Role

Use nursing process model following pre-, intra-, and posttest care guidelines in Chapter 1. See page 8 for list of appropriate nursing diagnoses.

Nursing Diagnosis

- Knowledge deficit related to lack or misinterpretation of information provided about purpose, procedure, and radiopharmaceutical injection and risk.
- High risk of injury/radiation hazard related to injection of radiopharmaceutical.
- High risk of infection related to venipuncture of radiopharmaceutical.

Pretest Care

◊ A signed, witnessed consent form must be obtained for heart shunt and exercise tests.
◊ See Nuclear Medicine Scans: Overview

• Explain purpose and procedure which will last about 1 hour. Fast at least 2 hours before test. No smoking. Reassure that radiopharmaceuticals are safe, have minimal side effects (nausea), and provide only minimal levels of radiation exposure. No metal objects on patient during testing. See alphabetical listing for Nuclear Scans, Overview. Test is contraindicated in pregnancy. Obtain an accurate patient weight.

Intratest Care

• During injection of radiopharmaceuticals, care may be needed for vertigo, nausea, and vomiting. Special nursing intervention and monitoring may be necessary for patients who have breathing difficulties and need certain medications and fluids. Perfusion tests with ^{99m}Tc require a light, fatty meal between rest and stress. Eight ounces milk are given 15 minutes after injection. Many tests require no eating during lengthy wait periods. Check with your lab.

Posttest Care

• Evaluate test outcomes; provide support and counseling as required. Biological excretions can undergo routine disposal unlesss patient is receiving radiation therapy. No prolonged contact for pregnant staff and visitors for 24–48 hours after radiation administration.
• Assess IV sites for signs of infection and adverse short-term effects of DPY (nausea, vomiting, headache, dizziness, facial flush, angina, ST segment depression, and ventricular arrythmia).
• Document any patient problems that may have occurred during and after procedure.

Heart Sonogram—
(Heart Echogram,
Echocardiography,
Echocardiogram,
Doppler Echocardiogram)

This noninvasive procedure visualizes cardiac structures as well as providing hemodynamic information regarding cardiac physiology.

Indications
• Evaluation of congenital cardiac abnormalities.
• Evaluate valve dysfunction and disease; abnormalities of blood flow; systemic and pulmonic hypertension.
• Evaluate myocardial disease.

Expected Test Outcomes
Normal position, size, and movement of heart valves and chamber walls. Appropriate blood flow and hemodynamic patterns.

Test Outcome Deviations
• Valvular disease: stenosis, prolapse dysfunction, function of prosthetic valves, pericardial effusion, tamponade, structural deformities, (congenital and acquired), and aneurysms.
• Myocardial dysfunction, hemodynamic disturbances, and cardiac lesions: tumors, thrombi.

Interfering Factors
• Dysrhythmias; hyperinflation of lungs with mechanical ventilation will obscure visualization of cardiac anatomy. Marked obesity, chest trauma, and dressings may adversely affect exam outcomes.

Procedure
• A specific clinical diagnosis (eg, evaluate mitral stenosis) should accompany the request for the test.
• A coupling medium, generally a gel, is applied to exposed chest in order to promote transmission of sound. A hand-held transducer is positioned on the chest between the ribs for this study. Electrocardiogram (ECG) may be attached to obtain tracings.

Nursing Role

Use nursing process model following pre-, intra-, and posttest care guidelines in Chapter 1. See page 8 for list of appropriate nursing diagnoses.

Nursing Diagnosis

- Knowledge deficit related to lack or misinterpretation of information provided about procedure and its purpose.
- Anxiety and fear related to unfamiliarity with diagnostic procedure and equipment.
- Ineffective coping related to test outcome and inability to accept diagnosis of cardiac disease.
- Decisional conflict related to test outcome and potential for interventional procedures.

Pretest Care

- Explain exam purpose and procedure. Assure patient that no radiation is employed and that test is painless. Typical exam time is 30–45 minutes.
- No preparation is necessary.
- Explain that a coupling gel will be applied to skin. Although couplant does not stain, advise patient to avoid wearing non-washable clothing.

Posttest Care

- Remove or instruct patient to remove any residual gel from skin.
- Evaluate patient outcomes; provide support and counseling.

••••••••••••••
CLINICAL ALERT

◇ Echocardiograms cannot be effectively performed over open wounds or dressings. Alternative methods such as transesophageal echocardiography (TEE) may be indicated.
••••••••••••••

Hematocrit (HCT); Packed Cell Volume (PCV)

See Complete Blood Count (CBC)

Hemoglobin (Hgb)

See Complete Blood Count (CBC)

Hemoglobin S (Sickle Cell Test)

See Sickle Cell Tests

Hepatitis Tests, HAV, HBV, HCV, HDV, HEV

Blood

These tests are done to diagnose viral hepatitis. Viruses known to cause hepatitis are referred to by letters: A, B, C, D, and E. Several tests are available for hepatitis testing and each test measures a specific antigen or antibody.

Indications

- Evaluate patients with jaundice and other symptoms of hepatitis.
- Aid in differentiation of various types of viral hepatitis, which is difficult because symptoms are similar.
- Evaluate blood products that have been donated for transfusion.

Procedure

- Serum (5 mL) obtained by venipuncture according to specimen collection guidelines in Chapter 2.

Expected Test Outcomes

Negative for hepatitis A, (HAV); B, (HBV); C (HCV); and D, (HDV).

Test Outcome Deviations

Appearance of Hepatitis Viral Markers Following Infection

SEROLOGICAL MARKER	TIME AFTER INFECTION	CLINICAL IMPLICATIONS
Hepatitis A virus (HAV)		Transmitted enterically; positive for acute state hepatitis A
HAV-Ab/IgM	4–6 wk	Develops early in disease, within 3–6 months.
HAV-Ab/IgG	8–12 wk	Indicative of previous exposure and immunity to hepatitis A.

(cont'd.)

SEROLOGICAL MARKER	TIME AFTER INFECTION	CLINICAL IMPLICATIONS
Hepatitis B virus (HBV)		Positive for acute stage hepatitis B
HBsAg-hepatitis B surface antigen	4–12 wk	Earliest indicator of presence of acute infection; also indicative of chronic infection
HBeAg	4–12 wk	Positive for acute active stage with viral replication (infectivity factor); "highly infectious."
HBcAB, hepatitis B core antibody	6–14 wk	This marker may stay in serum for longer time and, together with HBsAB, represents convalescent stage; indicates past infection.
ABcAbIgM	6–14 wk	Indicates acute infection.
HBeAb antibody	8–16 wk	Indicates resolution of acute infection.
HbsAb antibody	4–10 mos	Indicative of previous exposure and immunity to hepatitis B, but not necessarily to other types of hepatitis; this is the marker for *permanent immunity*.
Hepatitis C virus (HCV) anti-HCV Formerly non-A–non-B		Transmitted through blood and body fluids. All possible routes have not been identified.
Hepatitis D virus (HDV) anti-HDV		Can only cause infection in presence of active HBV infection.
Hepatitis E virus (HEV) No tests yet available.		Transmitted enterically.

Interfering Factors

- Present methods of testing for hepatitis virus markers are not sensitive enough to detect all possible cases of hepatitis.

Nursing Role

Use nursing process model following pre-, intra-, and posttest care guidelines in Chapter 1. See page 8 for list of appropriate nursing diagnoses.

Nursing Diagnosis

- Knowledge deficit related to lack of information or misinterpretation of information provided about purpose, procedure, and meaning of test outcomes.
- High risk of injury or infection related to venipuncture.

Pretest Care

- Assess patient's knowledge of test and clinical symptoms, and explain purpose and blood test procedure. Advise patient that enteric, blood, and body fluid precautions will be followed until results of hepatitis testing are available.

Posttest Care

- Evaluate patient outcomes and counsel appropriately. Provide information for patient regarding precautions needed to avoid transmission of virus to others. Continue precautions to avoid transmission of virus if test results are positive.

Histoplasmosis Test

See Fungal Antibody Test

HIV Test

SeeAntibody to Human Immunodeficiency Virus Test

Holter Continuous EKG Monitoring   Special Study

Holter monitoring records a continuous heartbeat for 24–48 hours or longer, by means of a portable recording device attached to the patient; concurrently keeps a diary of symptoms and activity status and pushes an event-marker button on the recorder to signal occurrence of symptoms.

Indications

- Document dysrhythmias and evaluate chest pain or other symptoms such as syncope, palpitations, dyspnea, or lightheadedness.

- Evaluate cardiac status after acute myocardial infarction or pacemaker implantation, and evaluate effectiveness of drug therapy.

Expected Test Outcomes

Normal cardiac rhythms.

Test Outcome Deviations

- Cardiac dysrhythmias such as premature ventricular contractions, conduction defects, tachyarrhythmias, brady-arrhythmias, and brady-tachyrhythmia syndrome.
- Hypoxic/ischemic changes.

Interfering Factors

- Smoking, eating, postural changes, certain drugs; Wolfe-Parkinson-White syndrome, bundle branch blocks, myocarditis, myocardial hypertrophy; anemia, hypoxemia, or abnormal hemoglobin binding can produce ST segment changes on the EKG tracing.
- Incomplete diary or failure to "mark" symptoms.
- Interference with electrode placement and adhesion.
- Changes in normal daily routines/activities.

Procedure

- Apply electrodes and attach electrode wires to monitor and recorder pack. Make sure everything is securely attached and that recorder has fresh batteries if necessary before calibrating and turning on.
- After monitoring period is completed, tape and diary are analyzed for patterns and variations in heart rhythm. The diary provides evidence of possible correlation between symptoms and results.

Nursing Role

Use nursing process model following pre-, intra-, and posttest care guidelines in Chapter 1. See page 8 for list of appropriate nursing diagnoses.

Nursing Diagnosis

- Knowledge deficit related to lack or misinterpretation of information provided about purpose and procedure.
- Anxiety related to test outcome and potential diagnosis of heart disease.

• Potential for noncompliance related to keeping of diary and event markers.

Pretest Care

• Explain purpose and procedure to patient. Demonstrate how equipment may be handled or attached to body.
• Encourage continuation of normal activities and emphasize diary entries related to activities, symptoms. Loose-fitting clothing that opens in front is best. Only sponge baths are allowed. Use care to keep electrodes dry.
• Record time monitor is started.

Posttest Care

• Record time monitor is discontinued.
• Cleanse electrode sites with mild soap and water and dry thoroughly.

....
CLINICAL ALERT

◊ Avoid magnets, metal detectors, high-voltage environments, and electric blankets.
◊ "Itching" under electrodes is common. Do not readjust placement sites.

....

Human T-Cell Lymphotrophic Virus-I (HTLV) Antibody

Blood

This test detects the presence of antibody to the human T-cell lymphocyte virus Type I (HTLV-I), a retrovirus associated with adult T-cell leukemia and demyelinating neurologic disorders.

Indications

• Evaluate patients with clinical diagnosis of adult T-cell leukemia.
• Evaluate patients who have been exposed to the blood of HTLV-I infected persons either through transfusion or sharing of needles for drug use.
• Screen persons whose blood and plasma products are being donated for transfusion.

Procedure

• Serum is obtained by venipuncture following specimen collection guidelines in Chapter 2.

Expected Test Outcomes

Negative for antibody to HTLV-I.

Test Outcome Deviations

• Positive results suggest infection with HTLV-I; repeatedly positive tests should be confirmed by Western Blot. HTLV-I infection has been confirmed in persons with adult T-cell leukemia, IV drug users, and healthy persons.

Nursing Role

Use nursing process model following pre-, intra-, and posttest care guidelines in Chapter 1. See page 8 for list of appropriate nursing diagnoses.

Nursing Diagnosis

• Knowledge deficit related to lack or misinterpretation of information provided about purpose, procedure and meaning of test outcomes.
• High risk of injury or infection related to venipuncture.

Pretest Care

• Assess patient's knowledge of test.
• Explain purpose and blood test procedure.

Posttest Care

• Advise patient, if test result is positive, that HTLV-I does not cause AIDS and the finding of HTLV-I antibody does not imply infection with HIV or a risk of developing AIDS.
• Provide counseling for patient to minimize anxiety associated with positive test results.

5-Hydroxyindoleacetic Acid (5-HIAA)(5-Hydroxy-3-Serotonin, Indoleacetic Acid)   Timed Urine

This test is conducted to diagnose a functioning carcinoid tumor, which is indicated by significant elevation of 5-HIAA, a denatured product of serotonin.

Indications

• Diagnose carcinoid tumors, low grade malignancies in appendix or intestinal wall.

Expected Test Outcomes

Quantitative: 3–15 mg/24 h or 10.4–41.6 µmoL/24 h.

Test Outcome Deviations

- *Levels over* 100 mg/24 h are indicative of large carcinoid tumor, especially when metastatic.
- *Increased levels* found in celiac disease, Whipple's disease, severe pain of sciatica or skeletal and smooth muscle spasm, cystic fibrosis, oat cell cancer of bronchus, bronchial adenoma of carcinoid type, and chronic intestinal obstruction.
- *Decreased levels* found in depressive illness, small intestinal resection, mastocytosis, phenylketonuria (PKU), Wartnup's disease.

Interfering Factors

- False positives can result if bananas, pineapples, plums, walnuts, eggplant, tomatoes, and avocados are eaten, as they contain serotonin.
- False positives can result with drug use: phenacetin, salicylates, reserpine (serpasil), methamphetamine (Desoxyn).
- False negatives can result with drug use: imipramine (Tofranil), methyldopa (Aldomet), MAO inhibitors, promethazine (Phenergan), phenothiazines, heparin, and ACTH.

Procedure

- Collect urine for 24 hours in clean container; may need acid preservative (pH < 4.0). See timed specimen collection guidelines in Chapter 2.
- Note drugs patient is taking on lab slip or computer screen.
- See Appendix E for standards of timed urine collection.

Nursing Role

Use nursing process model following pre-, intra-, and posttest care guidelines in Chapter 1. See page 8 for list of appropriate nursing diagnoses.

Nursing Diagnosis

- Knowledge deficit related to lack or misinterpretation of information provided about purpose and procedure of timed urine collection.
- Potential for noncompliance to test protocols related to high anxiety, confusion, denial.

Pretest Care

- Assess patient compliance and knowledge base prior to explaining test purpose and procedure.
- Patient should take no drugs for 72 hours before test if at all possible, and should not eat foods listed 72 hours before test.

Intratest Care

- Accurate test results depend upon proper collection, preservation, and labeling. Be sure to record test start and completion times.
- Food and water are permitted but foods high in serotonin content are not to be eaten during test.

Posttest Care

- Evaluate patient outcome. Provide counseling and support as appropriate.

Immune Function Tests   Blood and Urine

Immunoglobulins (IgG, IgA, and IgM), Immunofixation
Electrophoresis (IFE), Monoclonal Protein,
T and B Cell Lymphocyte Counts and Ratio; T-Helper,
T-Suppressor Ratio, C_3, C_4 Complement

These tests measure immune status and competence by identifying specific cells, immunoglobulins, and complements involved in the immune response.

Indications

- Investigate history of repeated infectious immune complex disorders, multiple myeloma, and other myeloproliferative disorders.
- Evaluate severity of nephritis, liver disease; diagnose and classify lymphocytic leukemia.
- Assess connective tissue disorders and lupus systemic erythematosus.
- Use T and B cell markers to assess immune status of HIV patients and monitor renal, bone marrow, and heart transplants.
- Monitor effectiveness of therapy through repeat testing.

Expected Test Outcomes

Immunoglobulins

TOTAL IGG (MEN AND WOMEN)

0–4 mos	141–930 mg/dL
5–8 mos	250–1,190 mg/dL
9–11 mos	320–1,250 mg/dL
1–3 y	400–1,250 mg/dL
4–6 y	560–1,308 mg/dL
7–9 y	598–1,379 mg/dL
10–12 y	638–1,453 mg/dL
13–15 y	680–1,531 mg/dL
16–17 y	724–1,611 mg/dL
>18 y	700–1,500 mg/dL

IGA (MEN AND WOMEN)

0–4 mos	5–64 mg/dL
5–8 mos	10–87 mg/dL
9–14 mos	17–94 mg/dL
15–23 mos	22–178 mg/dL
2–3 y	24–192 mg/dL
4–6 y	26–232 mg/dL
7–9 y	33–258 mg/dL
10–12 y	45–285 mg/dL
13–15 y	47–317 mg/dL
16–17 y	55–377 mg/dL
>18 y	60–400 mg/dL

IGM (MEN)

0–4 mos	5–64 mg/dL
5–8 mos	10–87 mg/dL
9–14 mos	17–94 mg/dL
15–23 mos	22–178 mg/dL
2–3 y	24–192 mg/dL
4–6 y	26–232 mg/dL
7–9 y	33–258 mg/dL
10–12 y	45–285 mg/dL
13–15 y	47–317 mg/dL
16–17 y	55–377 mg/dL
>18 y	60–400 mg/dL

IGM (WOMEN)

0–4 mos	14–142 mg/dL
5–8 mos	24–167 mg/dL
9–23 mos	35–242 mg/dL
2–3 y	41–242 mg/dL
4–17 y	56–242 mg/dL
>18 y	60–300 mg/dL

Monoclonal Protein

No abnormality.

T and B Surface Markers

Percent T Cells (CD2): 60%–88%

Percent Helper Cells (CD4): 34%–67%

Percent Suppressor Cells (CD8): 10%–42%

Percent B Cells (CD19): 3%–21%

Absolute Counts

Lymphocytes: 0.66–4.60 thou/μL

T Cells: 644–2201 cells/μL

Suppressor T Cells: 182–785 cells/μL

B Cells: 92–392 cells/μL

Lymphocyte Ratio	**C₃ Level**
TH/TS Ratio >1.0	75–150 mg/dL
	C₄ Level
	10–30 mg/dL

Test Outcome Deviations:
Immunoglobulins IgG, IgA, and IgM

- *IgG increases* occur in infections of all types, hyperimmunization, liver disease, malnutrition (severe), dysproteinemia, disease associated with hypersensitivity granulomas, dermatologic disorders, IgG myeloma, and rheumatoid arthritis.
- *IgG decreases* occur in agammaglobulinemia, lymphoid aplasia, selective IgG/IgA deficiency, IgA myeloma, Bence-Jones proteinuria, and chronic lymphoblastic leukemia.
- *IgA increases* occur in chronic, nonalcoholic liver diseases, especially primary biliary cirrhosis (PBC); PBC is a progressive disease most commonly seen in women in the second half of their reproductive period. Increases also occur in obstructive jaundice, a wide range of conditions that affect mucosal surfaces, during exercise, with alcoholism, and in subacute and chronic infection.
- *IgA decreases* occur in ataxia-telangiectasia, chronic sinopulmonary disease, congenital deficit, late pregnancy, prolonged exposure to benzene, abstinence from alcohol after a period of 1 year, immunosuppressive therapy protein-losing gastroenteropathies, and immunologic deficiency states.

· · · · · · · · · · · · ·
CLINICAL ALERT

◊ Persons with IgA deficiency are predisposed to autoimmune disorders and can develop antibody to IgA with possible anaphylaxis occurring if transfused.
◊ In the newborn, a level of IgM above 20 mg/dL is an indication of in utero stimulation of the immune system and stimulation by the rubella virus, the cytomegalovirus, syphilis, or toxoplasmosis.
· · · · · · · · · · · · ·

- *IgM increases* in adults occur in Waldenstrom's macroglobulinemia, trypanosomiasis, actinomycosis, Carrion's disease (bartonellosis), malaria, infectious mononucleosis, lupus erythematosus, rheumatoid arthritis, and dysgammaglobulinemia (certain cases).
- *IgM decreases* occur in agammaglobulinemia, lymphoprolif-

erative disorders (certain cases), lymphoid aplasia, IgG and IgA myeloma, dysgammaglobulinemia, and chronic lymphoblastic leukemia.

Test Outcome Deviations: Monoclonal Protein

- *Monoclonal proteins* in multiple myeloma (99%), in serum, or urine. Macroglobulinemia of Waldenstrom is characterized by presence of a monoclonal IgM protein in the serum in all cases.
- A monoclonal light chain (Bence-Jones protein) is found in the urine of approximately 75% of patients with multiple myeloma. Approximately 75% of patients with Waldenstrom's macroglobulinemia will have a monoclonal light chain in the urine. Heavy-chain fragments as well as free light chains may be seen in the urine of patients with multiple myeloma or amyloidosis.

Test Outcome Deviations: T and B Cells

- *A decrease of B cells primary*: transient hypogammaglobulinemia of infancy and X-linked hypogammaglobulinemia, selective deficiency of IgG, IgA, IgM; *secondary*: lymphomas, nephrotic syndrome, and multiple myeloma.
- *Decrease in T-cells primary*: DeGeorge's syndrome and Nezelot's syndrome; *secondary*: Hodgkin's or other malignant diseases, and acute viral infection such as measles (transient decrease).
- *Combined decrease in B and T cells primary*: autosomal or sex-linked recessive cause, Wiskott-Aldrich syndrome, and immunodeficiency with ataxia and telangiectasis; *secondary*: radiation and aging.
- *T cells increase* in Graves' disease, and *B cells increase* in active lupus erythematosus and chronic lymphocytic leukemia.
- Standard immunosuppressive and cytotoxic drug therapy usually decreases lymphocyte totals.
- In AIDS, the T4/T8 ratio decreases (< 1) due to a loss of T-helper lymphocytes.

Interfering Factors (T and B Cell Markers)

- Improper performance and collection procedure will invalidate test results.
- Failure to perform test within 24 hours after time of collection will result in requesting a fresh sample and another venipuncture.
- If peripheral blood is refrigerated instead of kept at room temperature until test is performed, a new sample must be collected.

Test Outcome Deviations: C_3, C_4 Complement

- *Decreased* C_3 levels with severe recurrent bacterial infections due to C_3 homozygous deficiency, immune complex disease, and membrane proliferative glomerulonephritis.
- *Increased* C_3 levels in numerous inflammatory states as an acute-phase response.
- *Decreased* C_4 levels with acute systemic lupus erythematosus, early glomerulonephritis, immune complex disease, cryoglobulinemia, inborn C_4 deficiency, and hereditary angioneurotic edema.
- *Increased* C4 levels with a variety of malignancies.

••••••••••••••
CLINICAL ALERT

◊ Patients with low C_3 levels are in danger of shock and death.
••••••••••••••

Interfering Factors (C_3)

- Specimen will produce a "falsely low" result if not processed properly—freeze serum within 2 hours from patient collection time.

Procedure (Immunoglobulins)

- Serum (10 mL) obtained from an adult by venipuncture according to specimen collection guidelines in Chapter 2.
- If test is requested on a child, a venous blood sample of 4–5 mL should be obtained. Minimum amount of serum needed to perform quantitative immunoglobulins on a pediatric sample is 0.5 mL serum.
- Check with individual lab performing test to see if fasting is required and to verify sample requirements.

Procedure (Immunofixation Electrophoresis, IFE)

- Serum (10 mL) obtained by venipuncture according to specimen collection guidelines in Chapter 2.
- Age of patient should be noted because IFE procedure is seldom indicated in patients less than 30 years of age. Monoclonal proteins are rarely identified in this age group.
- Submit 25 mL from a 24-hour urine collection if a urine IFE is to be run simultaneously. Again, patient's age should be noted on lab slip or computer screen. For IFE, follow 24-hour urine specimen collection guidelines in Chapter 2. Random urine sample for IFE may also be ordered. Collect specimen

per guidelines in Chapter 2.
• See Appendix E for standards of timed urine collection.

Procedure (T and B Cells)

• A venous blood sample (5–10 mL serum) with EDTA antico-agulant obtained by venipuncture according to specimen collection guidelines in Chapter 2. It should be delivered to laboratory as soon as possible so testing can be performed within 6 hours from time of collection (24 hour maximum).
• It is imperative that a separate 5–10 mL EDTA blood sample is collected for a CBC and differential to be performed. Pathologist's interpretation is based upon absolute values, not percentages of cell populations.
• Analysis is performed using a flowcytometer, an instrument which qualitatively and quantitatively measures peripheral blood cells.

Procedure C_3 and C_4

• Serum (at least 2 mL) obtained by venipuncture according to specimen collection guidelines in Chapter 2.
• Sample should be processed by lab within 2 hours from patient collection as C_3 is labile at room temperature and will be destroyed if serum is not frozen until test can be performed.

Nursing Role

Use nursing process model following pre-, intra-, and posttest care guidelines in Chapter 1. See page 8 for list of appropriate nursing diagnoses.

Nursing Diagnosis

• Knowledge deficit related to lack or possible misinterpretation of information provided about procedure and purpose.
• High risk of injury or infection related to venipuncture.
• Ineffective individual coping related to test outcomes and inability to accept need for repeat testing.

Pretest Care

• Verify patient's age, that a CBC and differential have been ordered, are collected from patient at some time as test for T and B cell lymphocyte markers. Be certain specimen is kept at room temperature and delivered to laboratory at once.
• Explain that these tests are used to screen for general immune

competence, provide base values, and to diagnose: C_3 (assess renal involvement of immune disorders); C_4 (assess SLE and RA); T and B cells (assess antibody)—produces B cells and T-helper lymphocytes to ward off bacterial and viral infections).

Posttest Care

- Evaluate patient outcomes and counsel appropriately.
- Prepare patient for possibility of repeat testing to determine if therapy is effective. For further characterization of monoclonal protein, a urine specimen may also be requested in addition to blood for serum protein electrophoresis (SPE) and IFE.
- If 24-hour urine collection is possible, make appropriate arrangements as timed is preferable to random urine.

Immunoelectrophoresis (IEP)

See Immune Function Tests

Immunoglobulins: IgG, IgA, and IgM

See Immune Function Tests

Infectious Mononucleosis Tests; Blood
Heterophile Antibody Titer Test;
Epstein-Barr Virus (EBV)
Antibody Tests

These tests measure heterophile antibodies and antibodies specific for Epstein-Barr virus (EBV) and are done in the investigation of infectious mononucleosis.

Indications

- Evaluate patients with clinical symptoms of infectious mononucleosis and atypical lymphocytosis.
- Differential diagnosis of chronic fatigue syndrome.

Expected Test Outcomes

Negative antibody titers.

Test Outcome Deviations

- Heterophile antibodies develop after first week or two of illness in 90% of symptomatic young adults. If heterophile test is negative in symptomatic individuals, tests for Epstein-Barr virus antibodies should be performed.

- Clinical symptoms disappear before abnormal blood results disappear.
- In chronic fatigue syndrome, EBV antibody levels stay elevated for length of the disease.

Interfering Factors

- 90% of normal adults have antibodies to EBV antigens.
- Less than 30% of EBV-infected children under age of 2 display heterophile antibodies.

Procedure

- Serum (5 mL) is obtained by venipuncture according to specimen collection guidelines in Chapter 2.

Nursing Role

Use nursing process model following pre-, intra-, and posttest care guidelines in Chapter 1. See page 8 for list of appropriate nursing diagnoses.

Nursing Diagnosis

- Knowledge deficit related to lack or misinterpretation of information provided about purpose and procedure.
- Anxiety about meaning of test outcome and relationship to disease cause.
- High risk for injury or infection related to venipuncture.

Pretest Care

- Assess patient's knowledge of test and clinical symptoms. Explain purpose and blood test procedure.

Posttest Care

- Evaluate patient outcomes, monitor, and counsel appropriately. Advise patient of disease course, resolution of symptoms, and possible follow-up testing. There is no drug therapy for the virus.
- Resolution of infectious mononucleosis follows a common pattern: pharyngitis disappears within 14 days, fever within 21 days, lymphadenopathy within 28 days. Fatigue may persist for months.

Intravenous Pyelogram (IVP)— Excretory Urography Kidney X-Ray

X-Ray Imaging with Contrast

This x-ray examination is used to evaluate the anatomy of the kidneys, ureter, and bladder and indirectly demonstrate renal function following intravenous contrast media injection.

Indications
- Rule out renal masses, hydronephrosis, and calculi.
- Evaluate renal trauma and congenital disease.

Expected Test Outcome

Normal size, shape, location of urinary structures and normal renal function; generally kidneys should be visualized within 5 minutes after administration of contrast media.

Test Outcome Deviations
- Congenital deformities (number, size, location of urinary structures); calculi, hydronephrosis, masses (cysts, tumors, hematomas, abscess); renal size deviations; renal dysfunctions as suggested by delayed renal visualization; and prostate enlargement (male).

Interfering Factors
- Retained feces, barium and/or intestinal gas will obscure visualization of the urinary tract.
- Metallic objects which overlie area of exam and severe obesity will interfere with organ visualization.

Procedure
- A preliminary abdominal x-ray film (KUB) is taken with patient in a supine position. Iodine contrast media is injected, generally into the antecubital vein. Multiple x-rays of the abdomen are taken at timed intervals.
- After satisfactory visualization of the renal structures, patient is asked to void. In most cases, a post-void film of bladder region is performed. Total exam time is 45–60 minutes. Exam length may be increased if there is a physiologic delay which prevents rapid clearing of contrast by the kidneys.

Nursing Role

Use nursing process model following pre-, intra-, and posttest care guidelines in Chapter 1. See page 8 for list of appropriate nursing diagnoses.

Nursing Diagnosis

- Knowledge deficit related to lack or possible misinterpretation of information provided about procedure or purpose.
- High risk for injury related to iodine contrast administration.
- Anxiety and fear related to unfamiliarity with diagnostic procedure and equipment.
- Ineffective coping related to test outcome and inability to accept diagnosis of urinary disease.

Pretest Care

- Assess for test contraindications (pregnancy, sensitivity to iodine contrast agents, severe renal dysfunction), elevated BUN, creatinine, food, beverage consumed 90 minutes prior to contrast administration. See Appendix A for nursing standards regarding x-ray contrast administration.
- Explain exam purpose and procedure.
- No food or beverage is allowed for approximately 8 hours prior to study. Make certain that jewelry and metallic objects are removed from abdominal area.
- A bowel prep is usually necessary. This may consist of cleansing enemas and/or laxatives. Check protocol at institution performing the study.

Intratest Care

- Encourage patient to follow breathing and positional instructions. Instruct patient to breathe slowly and deeply during contrast administration.
- Observe closely for signs of allergic reaction (hives, respiratory distress, changes in blood pressure, convulsions). Local reactions such as redness and pain at injection site can be treated with warm compresses.

Posttest Care

- Provide plenty of fluids, food, and rest after study.
- Observe for evidence of reactions such as nausea, skin rashes, hives. Document and inform physician.
- Evaluate patient outcomes; provide support and counseling.

Iron Tests

Transferrin, Total Iron-Binding Capacity, Ferritin and Iron

These tests measure forms of iron storage in the body and are helpful studies of anemia.

Indications

- Evaluate iron deficiency and blood loss.
- Aid or differentiate diagnosis of anemias.
- Assess nutritional status.

Expected Test Outcomes

Transferrin: 240–480 mg/dL
Total iron-binding capacity (TIBC): 240–450 µg/dL
Ferritin
   Men: 18–270 ng/mL or µg/L
   Women: 18–160 ng/mL or µg/L
   Children: 7–140 ng/mL or µg/L
   Newborn: 25–200 ng/mL or µg/L
   1 month: 200–600 ng/mL or µg/L
   2–5 months: 50–200 ng/mL or µg/L
Iron
   Men: 70–175 µg/dL
   Women: 50–170 µg/dL

Test Outcome Deviations: Transferrin

- *Transferrin increases* in iron-deficiency anemia due to hemorrhage, acute and viral hepatitis, estrogen therapy, and contraceptives.
- *Transferrin decreases* in microcytic anemia of chronic disease, protein deficiency or loss, inflammatory states, liver and renal disease, and genetic deficiency.

Interfering Factors, Transferrin

- Age (elevated in 2 1/2–10 years) and 3rd trimester pregnancy and some drugs affect levels (chloramphenicol and fluorides).

Test Outcome Deviations: TIBC

- *TIBC increases* in iron deficiency anemia, oral contraceptives, pregnancy, blood loss, and acute liver damage.
- *TIBC decreases* in hypoproteinemia from malnutrition, hemo-

chromatosis, anemia with infection and chronic disease, liver cirrhosis, and nephrosis.

Test Outcome Deviations: Ferritin

- *Ferritin increases* in iron overload status, acute hepatitis, Gaucher's, malignancies, and chronic inflammatory disorders.
- *Ferritin decreases* in iron deficiency and depletion status.

Interfering Factors, Ferritin

- Recently administered radiopharmaceuticals for nuclear scans cause spurious results.

Test Outcome Deviations: Iron

- *Iron increases* (amount of transferrin-bound iron) in hemolytic anemias, lead poisoning, pernicious anemia, hemochromatosis, after transfusion and iron administration.
- *Iron decreases* in bleeding and in iron deficiency, inflammation, infection, tumor, or myocardial infarction.

Interfering Factors, Iron

- Iron levels may be 10 times as high in morning as at night.

Procedure

- Serum or plasma (2 mL) is obtained by venipuncture following specimen collection guidelines in Chapter 2.

Nursing Role

Use nursing process model following pre-, intra-, and posttest care guidelines in Chapter 1. See page 8 for list of appropriate nursing diagnoses.

Nursing Diagnosis

- Knowledge deficit related to lack of information or possible misinterpretation of information provided about procedure, equipment, purpose, and preparation.
- High risk for injury, bleeding, hematoma, or infection following venipuncture.

Pretest Care

- Explain purpose and procedure of test.

Posttest Care

- Evaluate patient outcomes, monitor, and counsel appropriately regarding iron-containing foods and possible bone marrow aspiration and biopsy, (the best and most reliable evaluation of total body iron status).

Ketones

See Urinalysis

17-Ketosteroids (17-KS)— 17-Hydroxycorticosteroids (17-OHCS)

Timed Urine

These tests of adrenal function measure the excretion of urinary steroids and are indicated in the investigation of endocrine disturbances of the adrenals and testes.

Indications

• Assess adrenocortical hormone function in men and women with signs and symptoms of related disorders.

Expected Test Outcomes

	17-KETOSTEROIDS (17-KS)	17-HYDROXYCORTICOSTEROIDS (17-OHCS)
Men	8–20 mg/24 h	3–10 mg/24 h
Women	5–15 mg/24 h	2–6 mg/24 h
Children	0–2 mg/24 h	
Elderly	4–8 mg/24 h	

Test Outcome Deviations

• *Increased 17-KS* in adrenal carcinomas, pregnancy (third trimester), premature infants, ACTH administration, testicular interstitial cell tumors, Cushing's syndrome, nonmalignant virilizing adrenal tumors, androgenic anhenoblastoma, luteal cell ovarian tumors, female pseudohermaphroditism, adrenogenital syndrome associated with adrenal hyperplasia and testosterone administration.
• *Decreased 17-KS* in Addison's disease, panhypopituitarism, myxedema, nephrosis, castration or eunuchoidism in men, general wasting disease, thyrotoxicosis, primary ovarian agenesis.
• *Increased 17-OHCS* in any acute illness or stress, Cushing's syndrome, adrenal adenoma, adrenal carcinoma, ACTH

therapy, severe hypertension, acromegaly, thyrotoxicosis.
• Decreased 17-OHCS in Addison's disease, general wasting disease, panhypopituitarism, hypothyroidism, cessation of ACTH therapy.

Interfering Factors

• Increased levels of ketosteroids and hydroxycorticosteroids are seen in severe stress and obesity.
• Increased levels of ketosteroids are present in the third trimester of pregnancy.
• Drugs which cause false positives include dexamethasone (Decadron), spironolactone (Aldactone), phenothiazines, ACTH, antibiotics.
• Drugs which cause false negatives include chlordiazepoxide (Librium), probenecid (Benemid), meprobamate (Miltown), estrogen, oral contraceptives, reserpine, promazine, quinidine, thiazide diuretics, prolonged use of salicylates.

Procedure

• Collect urine for 24 hours in a clean container. Keep refrigerated. An acid preservative is usually added to keep the urine at a pH of < 4.5. See timed specimen collection guidelines in Chapter 2 and Appendix E for standards regarding urine collection.
• List drugs patient is taking on lab slip or computer screen.

Nursing Role

Use nursing process model following pre-, intra-, and posttest care guidelines in Chapter 1. See page 8 for list of appropriate nursing diagnoses.

Nursing Diagnosis

• Knowledge deficit related to lack of or possible misinterpretation of information provided about procedure, purpose, preparation, and need for patient cooperation.
• Ineffective individual coping related to test outcome and inability to accept diagnosis of serious disease.
• Potential for noncompliance related to inability to adhere to test collection protocols.

Pretest Care

• Assess patient compliance and patient knowledge base prior to explaining test purpose and procedure.

- If female has her menstrual period, postpone the test. A false positive 17-KS could result.
- Drugs which could interfere with test should not be taken for 48 hours prior to test; check with physician.

Intratest Care
- Food and fluids are permitted.
- Accurate test results depend on proper collection, preservation, and labeling. Be sure to include test start and completion times.

Posttest Care
- Evaluate patient outcome. Provide counseling and support as appropriate.

Kidney Function Tests   Blood and Urine

Blood Urea Nitrogen (BUN), Creatinine, Uric Acid, Osmolality

These tests are done to measure kidney function, diagnose renal failure and kidney disease, and aid in kidney dialysis management.

Indications
- Assess creatinine as index of kidney disease and before administering nephrotoxic chemotherapy.
- Measure BUN as index of glomerular function as well as production and excretion of urea. Check BUN in persons who are confused, disoriented, or convulsing.
- Measure uric acid to evaluate renal failure, gout, leukemia, and toxemia of pregnancy.
- Measure osmolality to evaluate concentration, hydration, antidiuretic hormone (ADH), and toxicology workup.

Expected Test Outcomes
BUN
   Adult: 7–18 mg/dL or 2.5–6.4 mmol/L
   Child: 5–18 mg/dL or 1.8–6.4 mmol/L
Creatinine
   Adult: 0.4–1.5 mg/dL; 3–18 y: 0.1-1.2 mg/dL; 0–3 y: 0.1-0.6 mg/dL

Uric acid
  Men: 3.5–7.2 mg/dL or 0.21–0.42 mmol/L
  Women: 2.6–6.0 mg/dL or 0.154–0.35 mmol/L
  Children: 2.0–5.5 mg/dL or 0.12–0.32 mmol/L
  Older Adult: Slightly increased
Osmolality, serum
  Adult: 275–295 m/Osmol/kg
  Newborn: as low as 266 m/Osmol/kg
Osmolality, urine
  Random: 50–1200 m/Osmol/L
  After 12-h fluid restriction: > 850 m/Osmol/L
  Ratio of serum/urine osmolality: 1.0–3.0

Test Outcome Deviations: BUN

- *BUN increases* (azotemia) in impaired renal function, shock, dehydration, diarrhea, diabetes, ketoacidosis, acute myocardial infarction congestive heart failure, severe crushing injuries, overwhelming infection, and excessive protein intake.
- *BUN decreases* in liver failure and disease, negative nitrogen balance (malnutrition and overhydration), impaired absorption as in celiac disease, among others.

Interfering Factors, BUN

- Decreases in diet (low protein and high carbohydrate), persons with smaller muscle mass, early pregnancy, and many drugs.
- Increases in late pregnancy, older adults, and many drugs.

Test Outcome Deviations: Creatine

- *Creatinine increases* in impaired renal function, nephritis, urinary tract obstruction, muscle disease, congestive heart failure, shock, and dehydration.
- *Creatinine decreases* not clinically significant occur in short stature, decreased muscle mass, and some abnormal liver disease.

Interfering factors, Creatinine

- Increases with ascorbic acid, many drugs and high meat diet.

Test Outcome Deviations: Uric Acid

- *Uric acid elevated levels (hyperuricemia)* in renal failure, gout, leukemia and cancers, acute infectious mononucleosis, severe eclampsia, shock, alcoholism, psoriasis, acidosis, diabetic ketosis, lead poisoning, polycythemia, hemoglobinopathies, and Down syndrome.

• *Uric acid decreased levels (hypouricemia)* after treatment with uricosuric drugs (allopurinol, probenecid, and sulfinipyrazone) and Fanconi syndrome, neoplastic disease (occasionally, Hodgkin's and some carcinomas), Wilson's disease.

Interfering Factors, Uric Acid

• Stress, fasting, and violent exercise will cause increases.
• Many drugs (long-term use of diuretics) and foods may affect levels.

Test Outcome Deviations: Osmolality

• *Osmolality increased* (hyperosmolality) with water restriction or loss, brain trauma, cerebral lesions, hypercalcemia, diabetes mellitus and diabetes insipidus.
• *Osmolality decreased* (hypo-osmolality) with loss of sodium with diuretics and low salt diet, Addison's disease, adrenogenital syndrome, inappropriate secretions of ADH as in trauma and cancer of lung, and excessive water replacement.

Interfering Factors, Osmolality

• Decreases with attitude, diurnal variation with water retention at night, and some drugs. Some drugs will cause increases.

Procedure

• Serum (6 mL) obtained by venipuncture according to specimen collection guidelines in Chapter 2. No fasting required.
• List patient drugs on laboratory slip or computer screen.
• Random morning urine specimen collected for osmolality after restricted fluids for 8–12 hours and high protein diet for 3 days. First voided morning specimen is not used. A second specimen taken about 2 hours later is collected and sent to laboratory. Follow collection guidelines in Chapter 2 for blood and urine specimens.
• See Appendix E for standards of timed urine collection.

Nursing Role

Use nursing process model following pre-, intra-, and posttest care guidelines in Chapter 1. See page 8 for list of appropriate nursing diagnoses.

Nursing Diagnosis

- Knowledge deficit related to lack or misinterpretation of information provided about purpose and procedure of kidney function tests.
- High risk of injury or infection related to venipuncture.
- Anxiety or fear related to negative test outcome and possibility of kidney disease diagnosis.
- Potential for noncompliance related to patient's ability to adhere to test requirements.

Pretest Care

- Explain purpose and procedure of test. In chronic renal disease, BUN correlates better with symptoms of uremia than does serum creatinine.

Posttest Care

- Evaluate patient outcome and monitor appropriately. With elevated BUN levels, fluid and electrolytes may be impaired. Notify physician of panic value of BUN greater than 100 mg/dL.
- A normal creatinine does not always indicate unimpaired renal function and cannot be used as a standard in known renal disease.

···············
CLINICAL ALERT

◊ Panic serum values for osmolality are results less than 240 or greater than 321. A value of 385 relates to stupor in hyperglycemia. Values of 400 to 420 are associated with grand mal seizures; values greater than 420 are deadly.

◊ The patient receiving intravenous fluids should have a normal osmolality. If osmolality increases, fluids contain relatively more electrolytes than water. If it falls, relatively more water than electrolytes is present. If ratio of serum sodium to serum osmolality falls below 0.43, the outlook is guarded. This ratio may be distorted in drug intoxication. Water-load or dilution test may be done to investigate impaired renal excretion of water.

◊ Panic value for creatinine is 10 mg/dL in nondialysis patient.
···············

Kidney Scan

See Renogram

Kidney Sonogram— Renal Ultrasound

Ultrasound Imaging

This noninvasive study is used to visualize the renal parenchyma and associated structures and is often performed following an intravenous pyelogram (IVP) to define and characterize mass lesions and/or the cause of a nonvisualized kidney.

Indications

- Differentiate obstructive from parenchymal renal disease.
- Characterize renal masses (cystic or solid) and infectious processes; visualize large calculi and detect ectopic or malformed kidneys.
- Guidance during biopsy, cyst aspiration, and other invasive procedures.
- Evaluate renal transplants.

Expected Test Outcomes

Normal sonographic image of renal parenchyma, collecting structures, blood vessels, and urinary bladder.

Test Outcome Deviations

- Presence of space-occupying lesions: cysts, solid masses and/or abscesses, hydronephrosis or other evidence of urinary tract obstruction; altered blood flow to/from kidney, and size, location, or structural abnormalities.

Interfering Factors

- Retained barium from prior radiographic studies may cause suboptimal results.
- Overlying intestinal gas, particularly in the case of a pelvic kidney, will obscure visualization.
- Obesity adversely affects tissue visualization.

Procedure

- A coupling medium, generally a gel, is applied to exposed abdomen in order to promote transmission of sound. A hand-held transducer is slowly moved across skin during

this imaging procedure. Patient is instructed to control breathing pattern while imaging is performed.
- Exam time is about 30 minutes. Both kidneys are routinely visualized.

Nursing Role

Use nursing process model following pre-, intra-, and posttest care guidelines in Chapter 1. See page 8 for list of appropriate nursing diagnoses.

Nursing Diagnosis

- Knowledge deficit related to lack of information or possible misinterpretation of information provided about procedure or purpose.
- Anxiety and fear related to unfamiliarity with diagnostic procedure and equipment.
- Ineffective coping related to test outcome and inability to accept diagnosis of renal disease.
- Decisional conflict related to test outcome and potential for interventional procedures.

Pretest Care

- Explain exam purpose and procedure. Assure patient that no radiation is employed and that test is painless.
- Limited preparation may be necessary. Some laboratories require patients to fast for 8–12 hours prior to procedure. Check with your ultrasound department for guidelines.
- Explain that a coupling gel will be applied to skin. Although couplant does not stain, advise patient to avoid wearing non-washable clothing.

Intratest Care

- Encourage patient to follow breathing and positional instructions.

Posttest Care

- Remove or instruct patient to remove any residual gel from skin.
- Evaluate patient outcomes, provide support and counseling.

··············
CLINICAL ALERT

◊ Scans cannot be effectively performed over open wounds or dressings.

◊ Exam must be performed before or more than 24 hours after barium administration.
◊ Patient must agree to and sign a surgical permit prior to performance of an ultrasound-guided biopsy or other interventional procedures.

....

_____

KUB (Kidneys, Ureter, Bladder)— Abdominal Plain Film, Flat Plate, Abdomen Series

X-Ray
Imaging

This x-ray study examines the area between the xiphoid and the pubic bones *without* the aid of contrast media.

Indications

• Rule out ascites, fluid collections, organ enlargement, rupture, calculi, masses, foreign bodies, and intestinal obstruction.
• Evaluate abdominal pain.
• Preliminary film prior to contrast studies, surgery.

Expected Test Outcomes

Normal abdominal structures.

Test Outcome Deviations

• Presence of space-occupying lesions such as calculi, foreign bodies, and tumors; abnormal size, shape, or position of intraabdominal organs; abdominal fluid collections such as ascites, and abnormal bowel patterns such as obstruction.

Interfering Factors

• Because retained barium will obscure abdominal structures, this procedure should be performed prior to any barium work.
• Severe obesity adversely affects image quality.

Procedure

• No fasting is required. Buttons, zippers, metallic objects should be removed from abdominal and back regions. Patient is asked to lie on his/her back on an exam table. Breathing may be suspended during x-ray exposure. Additional films may be taken with patient standing or lying on his/her side.

- The test is quick and painless.

Nursing Role

Use nursing process model following pre-, intra-, and posttest care guidelines in Chapter 1. See page 8 for list of appropriate nursing diagnoses.

Nursing Diagnosis

- Knowledge deficit related to lack or possible misinterpretation of information provided about procedure or purpose.
- Anxiety and fear related to unfamiliarity with diagnostic procedure and equipment.
- Ineffective coping related to test outcome and inability to accept diagnosis of disease.

Pretest Care

- Assess for test contraindications (pregnancy).
- Explain exam purpose and procedure. Assure patient that test is painless.
- No preparation is necessary. Make certain all jewelry and metallic objects are removed from abdominal area.

Intratest Care

- Encourage patient to follow breathing and positional instructions.

Posttest Care

- Evaluate patient outcomes; provide support and counseling.

Lactic Acid Dehydrogenase (LD, LDH)

See Cardiac Enzyme Tests

Laparoscopy— Pelviscopy, Peritoneoscopy

Endoscopic Imaging

Intraabdominal and pelvic cavities are examined and sometimes biopsied by means of laparoscopes or pelviscopes inserted through small incisions made into the anterior abdominal wall.

Indications

- Evaluate liver disease, portal hypertension, unexplained ascites, ovarian carcinoma, or for staging lymphomas or other abdominal masses.
- Evaluate advanced chest, gastric, pancreatic, endometrial, or rectal tumors.
- Diagnose cysts, adhesions, fibroids, malignancies, inflammatory process, infections, and infertility.

Expected Test Outcomes

- Gynecologic: uterus, ovaries, and fallopian tubes normal in size, shape, and appearance.
- Abdominal: liver, gallbladder, spleen, and greater curvature of stomach normal in size, shape, and appearance.

Test Outcome Deviations

- Endometriosis, ovarian cysts, pelvic inflammatory disease, carcinoma, metastatic sites, uterine fibroids, abscesses, hydrosalpinx, ectopic pregnancy, infection.
- Adhesions, ascites, cirrhosis, nodules, engorged vasculature (portal hypertension).

Procedure

- Protocols for local, spinal, or general surgery are followed. Puncture sites are made near the umbilicus and in other areas so that the scope and other instruments may access the operative site.
- Carbon dioxide or a non-conductive flushing solution (ex: glycerine) introduced into cavity causes organs and tissues to "push" out of the way so that better visualization and access are obtained.
- Access sites are closed with a few sutures or steri-strips and a small adhesive dressing is applied to the site.

Nursing Role

Use nursing process model following pre-, intra-, and posttest care guidelines in Chapter 1. See page 8 for list of appropriate nursing diagnoses.

Nursing Diagnosis

- Knowledge deficit related to lack or misinterpretation of information provided about purpose and procedure.

- Anxiety and acute pain related to effects of laparoscopy procedure.
- Ineffective airway clearance related to pain from operative area when coughing post-procedure.
- High risk for injury related to endoscopic procedure.

Pretest Care

- Explain test purpose and procedure; assess patient's knowledge level.
- Chart and check required lab tests and other diagnostic tests. Report abnormals to physician.

. . . .
CLINICAL ALERT

◇ Obtain properly signed and witnessed consent form.
◇ Patient must be in a fasting state from midnight before unless otherwise ordered. Carry out bowel prep if ordered.
. . . .

Posttest Care

- Recover patient according to protocols. Include frequent checks of vital signs and wounds.
- Administer pain medication as needed/ordered. Advise patient that shoulder and abdominal discomfort may persist for a few days; semi-Fowler's position and mild oral analgesics may reduce discomfort.
- Observe for hemorrhage, bowel or bladder perforation, or infection.
- If catheter has been removed, assess postop voiding within 8 hours.

. . . .
CLINICAL ALERTS

◇ These procedures may be contraindicated in persons with advanced abdominal carcinomas, severe respiratory or cardiac disease, intestinal obstruction, palpable abdominal mass, large hernia, tuberculosis, or history of peritonitis.
◇ Procedure may be interrupted in the event of massive bleeding or evidence of malignancy.
◇ Be alert for postop signs of bladder or bowel perforation or hemorrhage.
. . . .

Lead

This test detects and measures the amount of lead as an indication of lead poisoning.

Indications

- Screen for lead toxicity.
- Monitor response to chelation therapy.

Expected Test Outcomes

Blood: Less than 10 µg/dL for both children and adults.
Urine: Up to 125 µg/24 h probably not associated with any evidence of lead poisoning.

Test Outcome Deviations

- *Increased levels* with industrial exposure, lead plumbing, leaded gasoline, fumes from heaters, lead-based paint, unglazed pottery, batteries, lead containers used for storage, contaminated cans, drinking water, hobbies such as stained glass activities, lead dust that parents bring home to children on clothing.

Procedure

- Whole blood obtained by capillary puncture. 7–10 mL whole blood, serum, or plasma obtained by venipuncture according to collection guidelines in Chapter 2.
- A 24–hour urine may be requested for a quantitative test. Follow collection guidelines in Chapter 2 and see Appendix E for standards for urine specimen collection and handling.

Nursing Role

Use nursing process model following pre-, intra-, and posttest care guidelines in Chapter 1. See page 8 for list of appropriate nursing diagnoses.

Nursing Diagnosis

- Knowledge deficit related to lack of or possible misinterpretation of information provided about purpose and procedure.
- High risk of infection, injury, bleeding, or hematoma related to puncture procedures.
- Knowledge deficit related to test outcomes that reveal need for information about environmental lead sources, both at

home and work place, and possible repeat testing.

Pretest Care

- Assess knowledge base and explain purpose and procedure for collection of specimen.

Posttest Care

- Evaluate patient outcomes and monitor and counsel appropriately. Assess for signs and symptoms of lead poisoning: at 10 µg/dL decrease in RBC production in children and adults; above 30 µg/dL both children and adults have kidney disease; above 40 µg/dL reproductive problems occur; above 40 µg/dL in adults, results in memory loss, irritability, sleeplessness, muscle weakness, tremors, confusion, behavior changes, digestive symptoms (lead colitis, abdominal cramps), constipation and occasional bloody diarrhea; at 15 µg in children, results in developmental delays, behavior and learning disabilities.
- If levels high, monitor urinary output. If less than 25 mL/h, report to physician and provide fluids.
- Monitor medical treatment for remaining lead from body (chelation). Most often corrections are done through diet and minerals—calcium, zinc, and iron.
- Explain need for follow-up testing of blood, urine, hair, nails, or tissue biopsy for lead.
- Counsel affected patient regarding removal of lead source which may be state-mandated.

··············
CLINICAL ALERT

◊ Children absorb 50% of the lead they eat.
◊ Adults absorb 20% of the lead they eat.
··············

Lipase

See Pancreatic Function Tests

Lipoprotein

See Cholesterol Tests

Liver Function Tests

Blood and Timed Urine

Serum Glutamic Pyruvic Transaminase (SGPT) or Alanine Amino
Transferase (ALT), Gamma-Glutamine Transferase (GGT), Ammonia, Bilirubin, Alkaline Phosphatase (ALP) Urobilinogen

These measurements are done primarily to evaluate liver function and diagnose liver and bone diseases.

Indications

- Assess liver malfunction, detect alcohol-induced liver disease,
  hemolytic anemias, and hyperbilirubinemia in newborns.
- Evaluate progress of liver and pancreatic disease and
  response to treatment.
- Measure GGT in differential diagnosis of liver disease in children and pregnant women.

Expected Test Outcomes

There is a great deal of variation in reported values because of
lab methods used.

(ALT)(SGPT)

Women: 7–17 µ/L at 30° C
Men: 7–24 µ/L at 30° C
Children: 5–28 µ/L at 30° C

GGT

Women: 5–55 µ/L
Men: 5–85 µ/L

Bilirubin

Total < 1.6 mg/dL
Direct 1 month to adult:
  < 0.5 mg/dL

Ammonia

Neonate: 64–107 µ/mol/L
< 2 week: 56–82 µ/mol/L
Child: 21–50 µ/mol/L
Adult: 9–33 µ/mol/L

Alkaline Phosphatase (ALP)

AGE (Y)	MALE (U/L)	FEMALE (U/L)
0–4	145–320	145–320
4–7	150–380	150–380
7–10	175–420	175–420
10–12	135–530	135–530
12–14	200–495	105–420
14–16	130–525	70–230
16–20	65–260	50–130
20+	17–142	17–142

Urobilinogen, Urine

2-hour specimen: 0.1–1.0 Ehrlich units/2 h; 24-h specimen: 1–4 mg/24 h; Random: 0.1–1 Ehrlich unit/mL.

Test Outcome Deviations: ALT

- *ALT (SGPT) increases* in hepatocellular disease and hepatitis, cirrhosis, metastatic liver tumor, obstructive jaundice/biliary obstruction, pancreatitis, myocardial infarction, infectious mononucleosis, burns, delirium tremors.
- Although the AST level is already increased in acute myocardial infarction, the ALT does not always increase proportionately.

Interfering Factors, ALT

- Many drugs falsely increase levels (salicylates high or low levels).

⋯⋯⋯⋯⋯⋯
CLINICAL ALERT

◊ Persons with elevated ALT should not donate blood because there is a risk of hepatitis C developing in the blood recipient.

Test Outcome Deviations: GGT

◊ *GGT increases* in many liver diseases and biliary tract diseases, pancreatitis and pancreatic/liver cancers, other cancers, and use of alcohol, barbiturates, and phenacetins.
◊ GGT values are normal in bone growth and disorders, pregnancy, renal failure, and strenuous exercise.

Test Outcome Deviations: Ammonia

◊ *Ammonia increases* in many liver diseases, hepatic coma, severe heart failure, pericarditis, acute bronchitis, transient elevated in newborns (may be fatal), hemolytic disease of newborn, pulmonary emphysema, some leukemias, and Reye's syndrome.
◊ *Ammonia decreases* in hyperornithinemias.
⋯⋯⋯⋯⋯⋯
Interfering Factors, Ammonia

- Levels vary with protein intake, many drugs, and exercise causes increase.

Test Outcome Deviations: Bilirubin

- *Bilirubin increases* accompanied by jaundice is due to hepatic, obstructive or hemolytic causes, and prolonged fasting. A 48-hour fast produces a mean increase of 240% in healthy persons and 194% with liver dysfunction.

- *Bilirubin indirect (nonconjugate) increases* in hemolytic anemias, large hematomas, hemorrhage, pulmonary infarcts.
- *Bilirubin direct (conjugated) increases* in cancer of head of pancreas and choledocholithiasis.
- *Bilirubin direct and indirect increase* (with direct more elevated) in lymphoma, cholestasis secondary to drugs, cirrhosis, and hepatitis.

··············
CLINICAL ALERT

◊ Adult panic value >12 mg/dL; newborns, panic value >15 mg/dL; initiate exchange transfusion at once or mental retardation may result.
··············

Interfering Factors, Bilirubin

- Decreases due to sunlight, contrast medium 24 hours before test, high fat meal, foods, and drugs cause yellow hue in serum.

Test Outcome Deviations: ALP

- *Alkaline phosphatase (ALP) marked increases* in obstructive jaundice, cancer, abscesses of liver, and biliary and hepatocellular cirrhosis, moderate increases in hepatitis, infectious mononucleosis, and pancreatitis.
- *ALP increases* in bone disease (increased calcium bone deposits), marked increases in Paget's disease, metastic bone tumor, moderate increases in osteomalasis, rickets, and healing fractures.
- *ALP increases* in hyperparathyroidism, pulmonary and myocardial infarction, Hodgkin's, cancer of lung or pancreas, inherited hypophophatasia.
- *ALP decreases* in malnutrition, scurvy, hypothyroidism.

Interfering Factors, ALP

- Increases in many drugs, age (young growing children, pregnant women, postmenopausal, older adults), and after IV albumin for several days.

Test Outcome Deviations: Urobilinogen

- *Urinary urobilinogen* increased by any condition that causes increase in production of bilirubin and by any disease that

prevents liver from normally removing reabsorbed urobilinogen from portal circulation, whenever there is excessive
destruction of red blood cells as in hemolytic anemias, pernicious anemia, malaria; also, in infections and toxic hepatitis, pulmonary infarct, biliary disease, cholangitis, cirrhosis-
viral and chemical (chloroform, carbon tetrachloride),
congestive heart failure.

- *Urinary urobilinogen* decreased or absent when normal
amounts of bilirubin are not excreted into intestinal tract.
This usually indicates partial or complete obstruction of bile
ducts, such as may occur in cholelithiasis, severe inflammatory disease, cancer of the head of the pancreas, during
antibiotic therapy; suppression of normal gut flora may prevent breakdown of bilirubin to urobilinogen, leading to its
absence in the urine.

Interfering Factors, Urobilinogen

- Peak excretion occurs from noon to 4 PM and amount of urobilinogen subject to diurnal variation. Strong alkaline urine
shows a higher value and strongly acid shows a lower value.
Intake of foods such as bananas may affect test outcome.
- False negative results may be associated with high levels of
nitrates in wine. Drugs which cause false negatives include:
ascorbic acid, ammonium chloride, antibiotics. Drugs which
cause false positives include: sodium bicarbonate, cascara,
sulfonamides, phenothiazines, phenazopyridine (Pyridium),
methenamine mandelate (Mandelamine).

Procedures

- ALT and GGT procedure: serum (5 mL) nonhemolyzed
obtained by venipuncture following collection guidelines in
Chapter 2.
- Bilirubin procedure: before breakfast, serum (5 mL) nonhemolyzed obtained by venipuncture. Protect sample from
sunlight. No air bubbles or shaking of sample. If specimen cannot be examined immediately, store in refrigerator or in dark-
ness. In infants, blood can be collected from a heel puncture.
- Ammonia procedure: a fasting plasma sample (3 mL) obtained
by venipuncture. Sample is placed in iced container and examined within 20 minutes. Note all antibiotics on lab slip or computer screen because these drugs may lower ammonia. See
Appendix E for standards of timed urine collection.

Procedure, Urobilinogen

- General instructions of a 24-hour or 2-hour specimen are followed depending on what has been ordered. See specimen collection guidelines in Chapter 2. The 24-hour timed collection is best done from 1–3 PM or 2–4 PM. Collect without preservatives. Record total amount of urine volume. Protect from light. Test immediately. See Appendix E for standards for timed urine collection and handling.

Nursing Role

Use nursing process model following pre-, intra-, and posttest care guidelines in Chapter 1. See page 8 for list of appropriate nursing diagnoses.

Nursing Diagnosis

- Knowledge deficit related to lack of or misinterpretation of information provided about purpose and procedure.
- High risk of injury, bleeding, hematoma, or infection related to venipuncture.
- Ineffective individual coping related to test outcome and inability to accept diagnosis of serious liver disease.

Pretest Care

- Explain purpose and procedure of various liver function tests, assess for interfering factors, patterns of abnormal test outcomes are more useful than individual test outcome developments.
- Advise regarding fasting restrictions. See procedures. Water is permitted.

Intratest Care

- For urobilinogen, avoid exposure to light.
- Accurate test results depend upon proper collection, preservation, and labeling. Be sure to include test start and completion times.

Posttest Care

- Evaluate patient outcomes, monitor and counsel appropriately. Explain need for follow-up tests. Sometimes individual tests can be normal in proven specific liver disease and normal values may not rule out liver disease.
- In persons with impaired liver function, demonstrated by

increased ammonia, the level can be lowered by reducing protein intake and administering antibiotics to reduce intestinal bacteria.

Liver Scan   Nuclear Medicine Scan Imaging

This nuclear test is used to demonstrate the functions, anatomy, and size of the liver.

Indications
- Evaluate functional liver disease (cirrhosis and hepatitis) and investigate right upper quadrant pain.
- Search for site of metastatic disease and differential diagnosis of jaundice, and detect hepatic lesions for biopsy.
- Evaluate ascites, infarction due to trauma, and effects from radiation therapy.

Expected Test Outcomes
Normal liver size, shape, and position within the abdomen; normal size of cardiac impression on liver; normally functioning liver and reticuloendothelial system.

Test Outcome Deviations
- Abnormal patterns in cirrhosis, hepatitis, hepatomas, sarcoidosis, metastasis, cysts, infarcts, abscesses, hemangiomas, cancer, and adenomas.

Procedure
- Radiopharmaceutical (technetium labeled sulfur colloid) is injected intravenously.
- After administration of radiopharmaceutical, patient lies on his/her back; pictures are taken 360 degrees around the body.
- Entire study usually takes 60 minutes from injection to finish.

Nursing Role
Use nursing process model following pre-, intra-, and posttest care guidelines in Chapter 1. See page 8 for list of appropriate nursing diagnoses.

Nursing Diagnosis
- Knowledge deficit related to lack of or misinterpretation of

information provided about purpose, procedure, and injection of radiopharmaceutical.
- High risk for injury/radiation hazard related to nuclear scan procedure.

Pretest Care
- Obtain and record weight.
- Explain purpose and procedure. Reassure patient regarding safety of radiopharmaceutical. See Nuclear Medicine Scans: Overview.

Intratest Care
- Provide encouragement that test is proceeding normally.

Posttest Care
- Evaluate patient outcomes and counsel appropriately.
- Dispose of body fluids and excretions using routine procedures unless patient is also receiving therapeutic radiopharmaceuticals to treat disease.
- Advise pregnant staff and visitors to avoid prolonged contact for 24–48 hours after radioactive administration.

Lower Extremity Venous (LEV) Duplex Sonogram
Ultrasound Imaging

This noninvasive Doppler procedure is used to visualize and document blood thrombosis.

Indications
- Evaluate chronic leg swelling, stasis pigmentation, and leg pain.

Expected Test Outcomes
- Normal venous anatomy demonstrating spontaneous blood flow, phasicity of flow (flow patterns that respond to the patient's respiratory changes), augmentation (a rush of venous flow superior to compression of the vein), competence of valves, and nonpulsatile flow.
- Absence of thrombi or occlusive disease.

Test Outcome Deviations
- Venous thrombosis, obstruction, and incompetent valves.

Interfering Factors

- Marked obesity may adversely affect exam outcomes.

Procedure

- Patient is asked to lie on exam table with head slightly elevated and exposed leg turned slightly outward. Coupling gel is applied to leg. A hand-held transducer is maneuvered over blood vessels from groin region to area of the calf. During Doppler evaluation, an audible signal representing blood flow can be heard.
- Brief compression of the veins is performed at select intervals in order to evaluate vessel pathology. This may be uncomfortable for some patients.
- Both legs are examined for comparison. Exam time is approximately 30 minutes.

Nursing Role

Use nursing process model following pre-, intra-, and posttest care guidelines in Chapter 1. See page 8 for list of appropriate nursing diagnoses.

Nursing Diagnosis

- Knowledge deficit related to lack or possible misinterpretation of information provided about procedure and purpose.
- Ineffective coping related to test outcome and inability to accept diagnosis of vascular disease.
- Decisional conflict related to test outcome and potential for interventional procedures.

Pretest Care

- Explain exam purpose and procedure. Assure patient that no radiation is employed and that no contrast media is injected.
- Advise that a coupling gel will be applied to skin. Although couplant does not stain, advise patient to avoid wearing non-washable clothing.

Posttest Care

- Remove or instruct patient to remove any residual gel from skin.
- Evaluate patient outcomes; provide appropriate support and counseling.

Lung Scans/Ventilation, Perfusion

Nuclear Medicine
Scan Imaging

Two types of scans are done: ventilation, to assess ventilation proces; and perfusion, to assess pulmonary vascular supply.

Indications

• Diagnose pulmonary emboli and investigate chest pain and respiratory distress.

Expected Test Outcomes

Normal functioning lung; normal pulmonary vascular supply, and normal gases exchanged.

Test Outcome Deviations

• Abnormal ventilation and perfusion patterns indicate lung tumors and cancer, emboli, pneumonia, atelectasis, asthma, inflammatory fibrosis, and chronic obstructive pulmonary disease.

Interfering Factors

• False-positive scans occur in vasculitis, mitral stenosis, pulmonary hypertension, and when tumors obstruct a pulmonary artery with airway involvement.

Procedure

• The patient is asked to breathe radioactive gas (Krypton, Xenon, or aerosol technetium) for approximately 5 minutes through a closed, nonpressurized ventilation system. During this time, a small amount of radioactive gas will be administered into the system. Breath-holding will be required for a brief period some time during the examination.
• The perfusion scan immediately follows the ventilation study.
• Radioactive technetium is injected IV.

Nursing Role

Use nursing process model following pre-, intra-, and posttest care guidelines in Chapter 1. See page 8 for list of appropriate nursing diagnoses.

Nursing Diagnosis

• Knowledge deficit related to lack or misinterpretation of

information provided about purpose, procedure, and breathing of radioactive gas.
- High risk of injury/radiation hazard related to radiopharmaceutical administration.
- Fear and mistrust related to nuclear medicine scan procedure.

Pretest Care
- Obtain accurate weight. Explain purpose, procedure, and patient cooperation.
- Alleviate any fears the patient may have concerning nuclear medicine procedures. See Nuclear Medicine Scans; Overview.
- A record of a recent chest x-ray must be available.

Intratest Care
- Provide encouragement and support.
- The patient must be able to follow directions for breathing and holding his or her breath.

Posttest Care
- Evaluate patient outcomes and counsel appropriately.
- Dispose of body fluids and excretions in routine ways unless patient is also receiving therapeutic doses of radiopharmaceuticals to treat disease.
- Advise pregnant staff and visitors to avoid prolonged contact with patient for 24–48 hours after radioactive administration.

Lyme Disease Test   Blood

This test is used to diagnose Lyme disease and measures antibodies caused by the spirochete *Borrelia burgdorferi* spread by deer ticks.

Indications
- Evaluate infection with *Borrelia burgdorferi* in patients lacking classic lesions of erythema chronicum migrans.
- Diagnose infection in patients outside an endemic area to identify antibodies to *Borrelia burgdorferi*.

Expected Test Outcomes
IFA titer <1:256; ELISA: nonreactive to antibodies

Test Outcome Deviations

- *Elevated levels* in 50% of patients with early Lyme disease and erythema chronicum migrans. Elevated levels in most patients with later complications of carditis, neuritis, and arthritis. Elevated levels are seen in some patients in remission.
- IgM antibodies develop early in the disease and IgG antibodies are consistently detected later in the disease.

Interfering Factors

- Tests currently available have low sensitivity and specificity. False positives are seen in patients with antibodies to other spirochetes such as *Treponema pallidum*, the causative agent of syphilis, and in persons with high levels of rheumatoid factor.
- Asymptomatic individuals in endemic areas may have antibodies to *Borrelia burgdorferi*.

Procedure

- Serum (5 mL) obtained by venipuncture according to specimen collection guidelines in Chapter 2. A follow-up specimen may be required.
- Tests available include IFA, ELISA, and Western Blot.

Nursing Role

Use nursing process model following, pre-, intra-, and posttest care guidelines in Chapter 1. See page 8 for list of appropriate nursing diagnoses.

Nursing Diagnosis

- Knowledge deficit related to lack of or misinterpretation of information provided about purpose and procedure of test.
- High risk for injury or infection related to venipuncture.

Pretest Care

- Assess patient's knowledge of test, clinical symptoms, and travel history to endemic areas. Explain purpose and blood test procedure. No fasting is necessary.

Posttest Care

- Evaluate patient outcomes and counsel appropriately. Advise patient, if test results are not diagnostic, that repeat testing may be required. Tell patient that antibiotic therapy will be used to treat disease if test results are positive.

Lymphangiogram (Lymphangiography)

X-Ray Imaging with Contrast

In this x-ray examination, the very fine lymphatic channels are visualized after injection of an iodinated contrast agent.

Indications

- Evaluation for Hodgkin's disease, lymphoma.
- Staging of cancers.
- Evaluate extremity edema of unknown etiology.

Procedure

- Lymphatic vessels are cannulized following injection of a blue contrast between the fingers for the upper extremity and/or toes for the lower extremity. Under local anesthetic, a small incision is made at the site of best lymphatic visualization. Under extremely low pressure, an iodinated contrast media is injected into the lymphatic vessel. The infusion of contrast may take several hours. Initial films are taken of the extremities, and pelvic or shoulder girdle. The patient is instructed to return for more filming approximately 24 hours postinjection. The total exam time may be 4 hours or more, depending upon the ease of cannulization of the lymphatic vessel.

Expected Test Outcomes

Normal lymphatic vessels and nodes.

Test Outcome Deviations

- Lymphoma, metastic involvement of lymph nodes, and abnormal lymph vessels.

Interfering Factors

- Retained feces, barium, and/or intestinal gas will obscure visualization of the abdominal/pelvic lymphatics.
- Metallic objects which overlie the area of interest will interfere with organ visualization.
- Severe obesity adversely affects image quality.

Nursing Role

Use nursing process model following pre-, intra-, and posttest care guidelines in Chapter 1. See page 8 for list of appropriate nursing diagnoses.

Nursing Diagnosis

- Knowledge deficit related to lack of information or possible misinterpretation of information provided about the procedure or purpose.
- Anxiety and fear related to unfamiliarity with diagnostic procedure and equipment.
- Discomfort and pain related to lymphangiography procedure.
- High risk of injury or infection related to injection site and contrast medium.

Pretest Care

- Assess for test contraindications (pregnancy); explain exam purpose and procedure and make certain that jewelry and metallic objects are removed from abdominal area.

••••••••••••••
CLINICAL ALERT
◊ Obtain a signed, witnessed consent form.
◊ See Appendix A regarding contrast media precautions.
••••••••••••••

Intratest Care

- Provide support during cannulization process as some discomfort can be expected. This procedure may be extremely long and tiring to patient. Encourage patient to follow breathing and positional instructions during x-ray exposures.

Posttest Care

- Check vital signs for at least 24 hours. Administer analgesics if necessary.
- Provide fluids, food, and rest after the study.
- If ordered, elevate legs to prevent swelling.
- Check for complications at injection site.
- Evaluate patient outcomes, provide appropriate monitoring, support, and counseling.

••••••••••••••
CLINICAL ALERT
◊ Lymphangiography may be contraindicated in known contrast/iodine hypersensitivity, severe pulmonary insufficiency, cardiac disease, and advanced renal or hepatic disease.
◊ In rare instances, the contrast media may embolize to the lungs.
••••••••••••••

Lymphocytes

See Complete Blood Count (CBC)

Magnesium

See Electrolyte Tests

Magnetic Resonance Imaging (MRI, MR), (Brain, Spine, Limbs, Joints, Heart (Cardiac), Abdomen, Pelvis)—MR Angiography

Special Imaging with Contrast

This computer-based procedure provides physiological information and detailed views of fluid-filled soft tissues and uses a superconducting magnet and radiofrequency (RF) signals to cause hydrogen nuclei to emit their own signals.

Indications

- Differentiate diseased tissue from healthy tissue and study blood flow.
- Evaluate multiple sclerosis, Alzheimer's disease, spine and cord abnormalities, neoplasms throughout the body, joint pathologies, cardiac function, and vascular pathologies.

Expected Test Outcomes

- Normal soft tissue structure of brain; spinal cord and subarachnoid spaces, fat, muscles, tendons, ligaments, nerves, blood vessels and marrow of limbs and joints, normal heart structure, soft tissues of abdomen and pelvis.
- Normal size, anatomy, and hemodynamics of blood vessels.

Test Outcome Deviations

- *MRI of brain* demonstrates white matter disease (multiple sclerosis, infections, AIDS), neoplasms, ischemia, cerebrovascular accident, aneurysms, and hemorrhage.
- *MRI of spine* demonstrates disc herniation, degeneration, neoplasms (primary and metastatic), inflammatory disease, and congenital abnormalities.
- *MRI of limbs and joints* demonstrates neoplasms, ligament or tendon damage, osteonecrosis, and bone marrow disorders.
- *MRI of heart* (cardiac MRI) demonstrates abnormal chamber

size and myocardial thickness, tumors, congenital heart disorders, pericarditis, graft instabilities, thrombi, aortic dissection, and aneurysms.

- *MRI of abdomen and pelvis* demonstrates neoplasms and tumor
  stage of liver, pancreas, adrenals, spleen, kidneys, blood vessels, reproductive organs, and abnormalities of renal transplants.
- *MRI angiography* demonstrates aneurysms, stenosis, occlu-
  sions, graft patency, and vascular malfunctions.

Procedure

- Patient is positioned before couch is moved into tunnel-shaped
  gantry. (Gantry is narrow and may frighten some individuals.)
  Patient is assured that there is sufficient air to breathe and that
  will be monitored during entire procedure.
- In some instances, a non-iodinated venous contrast will be
  injected for better visualization of anatomy. The most commonly used contrast agent is gadolinium DTPA which has
  very low toxicity and much fewer side effects than iodine
  contrast agents. Gadolinium is generally used in examinations of the central nervous system (brain and spine). Exam
  time will vary between 60 and 90 minutes.

Nursing Role

Use nursing process model following pre-, intra-, and posttest
care guidelines in Chapter 1. See page 8 for list of appropriate
nursing diagnoses.

• • • • • • • • • • • • •
CLINICAL ALERT

◊ Safety concerns for patient and staff during MRI procedures
  are based upon interaction of strong magnetic fields with
  body tissues and metallic objects. These potential hazards are
  mainly due to *projectiles* (metallic objects can be displaced,
  giving rise to potentially dangerous projectiles); *torquing of
  metallic objects* (implanted surgical clips and other metallic
  structures can be torqued or twisted within the body when
  exposed to strong magnetic fields); *local heating* (exposure to
  RF pulses can cause heating of tissues or metallic objects
  within patient's body; for this reason, pregnant women are
  not routinely scanned since an increase in amniotic
  fluid/fetal temperature may be harmful); *interference with
  electromechanical implants* (electronic implants are at risk for
  damage from both magnetic fields and the RF pulses; conse-

quently, those with cardiac pacemakers, implanted drug infusion pumps, cochlear implants, and similar devices should not be exposed to MR procedures).

◊ In the event of a respiratory/cardiac arrest, patient is removed from the scan room prior to resuscitation. Most general hospital equipment (oxygen tanks, wheelchairs, IV pumps, and monitors) are not permitted in the MR suite.

◊ Absolute contraindications to MRI include:
1. Implanted devices including pacemakers, cochlear implants, some prosthetic devices (consult with MR lab for specific information), implanted drug infusion pumps, neurostimulators, bone growth stimulators, and certain IUCD (intrauterine contraceptive devices);
2. Internal metallic objects, including metallic fragments, bullets, shrapnel and surgical clips, pins, plates, screws, metal sutures, or wire mesh.

◊ In addition, MRI is generally not advised for the pregnant patient or individuals with epilepsy. All patients must remove the following materials prior to entering the MRI suite: hearing aids, dentures, jewelry, hair pins, wigs and hair pieces.

◊ Severely obese patients may not fit into the small gantry opening.

◊ Patients unable to hold still or who are claustrophobic may require conscious sedation prior to MRI procedures.

Nursing Diagnosis

• Knowledge deficit related to lack of information or possible misinterpretation of information provided about procedure and purpose.

• Anxiety and fear related to unfamiliarity with diagnostic procedure and equipment.

• Discomfort and claustrophobia related to MRI equipment.

• Decisional conflict related to test outcome and potential for interventional treatment.

Pretest Care

• Explain MRI purpose and procedure. Obtain patient history regarding contraindications to MR. See Clinical Alert. No pain is associated with MR.

• Sedation may be required if patient is claustrophobic or otherwise unable to lie still during procedure. Ear protection aids in eliminating "knocking" sound emanating from scanner. Patient is assured that a two-way communication system between patient and operator will allow for continual monitoring and vocal feedback.

Intratest Care
• Provide reassurance during testing.

Posttest Care
• Evaluate patient outcomes and counsel appropriately.

Mammography— Breast X-Ray
X-Ray Imaging

Mammography is an x-ray of the soft tissues of the breasts.

Indications
• Known or suspected breast mass, skin or nipple changes, and nipple discharge.
• Screening exam for breast disease in all women over the age of 35–40.

Expected Test Outcomes
Normal breast tissue.

Test Outcome Deviations
Masses, cysts, tumors, abscesses, and calcifications.

Procedure
• Patient is asked to identify any known lumps/lesions. A pertinent GYN and family history is usually taken. A physical breast exam may be performed.
• The breasts are exposed and positioned in a device used to compress the tissue. This brief compression will aid in visualization and will also reduce amount of radiation that needs to be applied to the breast. Generally, two images are made of each breast.
• Exam time is generally less than 30 minutes.

Nursing Role
Use nursing process model following pre-, intra-, and posttest care guidelines in Chapter 1. See page 8 for list of appropriate nursing diagnoses.

Nursing Diagnosis

- Knowledge deficit related to lack of information or possible misinterpretation of information provided about the procedure or purpose.
- Anxiety and fear related to unfamiliarity with diagnostic procedure and equipment and possible diagnosis of breast cancer.

Pretest Care

- Assess for test contraindications: pregnancy.
- Explain exam purpose and procedure. Some discomfort is to be expected during breast compression. Make certain that jewelry and metallic objects are removed from the chest area. Advise patient to refrain from using underarm deodorants prior to mammography as these may produce an image artifact. Instruct patient to wash breasts prior to exam. Most patients are most comfortable if they wear a two-piece outfit to the lab, which will allow easy removal of upper body clothing. Suggest that patients who have painful breasts refrain from coffee, tea, cola, and chocolate 5–7 days before the mammogram.

Posttest Care

- Evaluate patient outcomes, provide support and counseling.

Monocytes

See Complete Blood Count (CBC)

Neonatal Thyroxine (T_4)   Blood

This test measures thyroxine (T_4) activity in the newborn.

Indications

Screen for hypothyroidism after 24 hours of life, preferably within first week.

Expected Test Outcomes

1–5 days: >7.5 μg/dL; > 97 nmol/L
6 days: 6.5 μg/dL; >84 nmol/L
Reference range for newborn screening are laboratory dependent.

Test Outcome Deviations

- *Increased T_4 values in hypothyroidism.*
- *Alert limits*:
  1–5 days: ≤ 4.9 µg/dL
  6–8 days: ≤ 4 µg/dL
  9–11 days: ≤ 3.5 µg/dL
  12–120 days: ≤ 3 µg/dL
- 6–12% of infants with hypothyroidism will have normal screening results.

Procedure

- Obtain blood sample by skin puncture following specimen collection guidelines in Chapter 2. The circles of the filter paper must be completely filled. This is best done by placing one side of the filter paper against infant's heel and waiting for blood to appear on front side of paper and completely fill the circle.
- Air dry for 1 hour; fill in all requested information and send to laboratory immediately.

Nursing Role

Use nursing process model following pre-, intra-, and posttest care guidelines in Chapter 1. See page 8 for list of appropriate nursing diagnoses.

Nursing Diagnosis

- Knowledge deficit of parents related to purpose, procedure, and significance of test outcome deviations.
- Anxiety of parents related to test outcome.
- High risk for injury related to skin punctures.

Pretest Care

- Assess parent knowledge base prior to explaining test purpose and procedure.

Posttest Care

- Evaluate patient outcome. Notify physician and parents of positive results within 24 hours. Advise regarding need for follow-up neonatal thyroid stimulating hormone (TSH) if results are positive.

Neutrophils

See Complete Blood Count

Nuclear Medicine Scans—Overview

Nuclear scans allow for visualization of tissues that cannot be seen on a simple x-ray. Space-occupying lesions, especially tumors, stand out particularly well. Generally, these lesions are represented by areas of reduced activity (cold spots) as in liver scans, or by increased activity (hot spots) as in bone imaging. After administration of radioactive materials, these radiopharmaceuticals will distribute throughout organ tissues, depending upon their specificity and route of administration. Within these organs, the radioactive material shows distributions in normal tissue that differ from those in diseased tissue. The main imaging device that shows the distribution of the radiopharmaceuticals is a gamma camera. These cameras are capable of "photographing" static, dynamic, and whole body. Today these gamma cameras have achieved a third dimension through single photon emission computed tomography (SPECT) and visualize individual slices of organs.

Patients retain the radioactivity for relatively short periods of time. The radioactive energy will decay on its own, and some of it will be eliminated in urine and feces. The most common radioactive source, technetium, is virtually gone from the patient's body in 24 hours after administration. Other sources such as iodine, indium, and thallium take from 13 hours to 8 days to dissipate half of the energy. Patients need to know that once the energy has eliminated, they are no longer carrying the radioactivity. Regardless of the amount of radioactivity, a radiation hazard to the patient always exists. In all nuclear medicine procedures, the value and importance of the information gained must be weighed against the potential hazard of radiation to the patient.

- Inform the patient that the procedure is performed in department of nuclear medicine and that most procedures last about an hour.
- Have the patient appropriately dressed, usually in robe and slippers. It is important that there be no metal objects on the patient during the procedure.
- Inform the patient that qualified technologists will provide appropriate instructions and care throughout the procedure.
- Reassure the patient that radiopharmaceuticals are safe, have minimal side effects (such as nausea), and provide minimal levels of radiation exposure.

- Obtain an accurate patient weight since this is the basis for the dose of radiopharmaceutical to be administered.
- In general, signed consent forms are not required unless required by the FDA or if the patient undergoes physical stress.

···············

CLINICAL ALERT

◊ Nuclear medicine procedures are contraindicated in pregnancy.

···············

Obstetric Sonogram— OB Ultrasound, Fetal Age Determination

Ultrasound Imaging

This noninvasive procedure is used to visualize and document fetal, placental, and maternal structures and to estimate fetal age and weight.

Indications

- Confirm presence and position of intrauterine gestation and rule out ectopic pregnancy, clarify size/date discrepancy (large or small for dates), and rule out suspected fetal pathology; and assess maternal pathologies (fibroids, cysts).
- Guide for amniocentesis, chorionic villi sampling, invasive procedures.

Expected Test Outcomes

Normal fetal, maternal, and placental anatomy; fetal viability; adequate amniotic fluid volumes.

Test Outcome Deviations

- Absence of pregnancy, fetal demise, presence of fetal abnormalities, and presence of uterine or adnexal abnormalities.
- Fetal age that does not correspond to expected dates; multiple gestation; molar pregnancy; placental pathologies (previa, abruptio); deviations in amniotic fluid volumes (oligohydramnios, polyhydramnios); deviations in fetal growth: growth retardation, macrosomia, and evidence of fetal distress (lack of breathing and movement).

Interfering Factors

- Gas overlying pelvic structures in early first trimester may compromise ultrasound study. Obesity adversely affects ultrasonic visualization of tissues. Posterior placentas may be obscured by overlying fetal anatomy.

Procedure

- Woman lies supine with abdomen exposed during procedure. First and second trimester scans generally require patient to have a full bladder when scanning trans-abdominally. Scans performed to evaluate placental location also require a full bladder in most cases. Scans of first trimester pregnancy may be performed with a transvaginal approach. In this procedure, bladder is not full; a slim, lubricated transducer is inserted directly into woman's vaginal vault.
- A coupling medium, generally gel, is applied to exposed abdomen/pelvis in order to promote transmission of sound. A hand-held transducer is slowly moved across skin during this imaging procedure. Exam time is about 30–60 minutes.

Nursing Role

Use nursing process model following pre-, intra-, and posttest care guidelines in Chapter 1. See page 8 for list of appropriate diagnoses.

Nursing Diagnosis

- Knowledge deficit related to lack of or possible misinterpretation of information provided about procedure, purpose, and preparation.
- Decisional conflict related to test outcome and potential disease of fetus or termination of pregnancy.
- Ineffective coping related to test outcome and inability to accept diagnosis of fetal, placental, or maternal disorders.
- Discomfort related to very full bladder.

Pretest Care

- Explain exam purpose and procedure; no radiation is employed and test is painless. Emphasize test preparation. In most cases, a full-bladder study is performed which will require patient to consume approximately 32 ounces of clear fluid (preferably water) 1–2 hours prior to procedure. Patient is instructed not to void until examination is completed. Discomfort associated with a very full bladder is to be expected.
- Explain that a coupling gel will be applied to skin. Although couplant does not stain, advise patient to avoid wearing non-washable clothing.

Intratest Care

- Since maintenance of a distended bladder may be quite difficult, offer encouragement to patient. If supine hypotension syndrome is experienced, instruct patient to turn on her back and breathe slowly and deeply.

Posttest Care

- Remove or instruct patient to remove any residual gel from skin. Instruct patient to empty bladder frequently upon completion of full-bladder study.
- Evaluate patient outcomes, provide support and counseling as required.

Orthopedic X-Ray   X-Ray Imaging

Diagnostic x-ray studies can be performed on a certain bone or bony part such as patella or wrist.

Indications

- Rule out fracture (trauma).
- Detect masses, arthritis, or other bone/joint pathologies.

Expected Test Outcomes

Normal osseous and soft-tissue structures.

Test Outcome Deviations

- Traumatic changes (fractures, dislocations), degenerative changes (arthritis, osteoporosis, aseptic necrosis), bone tumors (benign, malignant, metastatic), osteomyelitis, abscess, infarcts, and osteochondrosis: eg, Osgood Schlatter, Legg-Calvé-Perthes.

Interfering Factors

- Jewelry, metallic objects, buttons, and other foreign bodies which may overlie the area to be studied will interfere with visualization of the bony part. Radiographic examination of the lower abdomen and pelvic region may be obscured due to retained barium.

Procedure

- Patient may be instructed to sit, lie on an exam table, or stand, depending upon body part being examined. Some manipulation of body part will occur in order to provide a minimum of two radiographic views. On occasion, restraints or other stabilizing hardware must be removed, requiring nursing assistance.

Nursing Role

Use nursing process model following pre-, intra-, and posttest care guidelines in Chapter 1. See page 8 for list of appropriate nursing diagnoses.

Nursing Diagnosis

- Knowledge deficit related to lack or possible misinterpretation of information provided about procedure or purpose.
- Anxiety and fear related to unfamiliarity with diagnostic procedure and equipment.
- Ineffective coping related to test outcome and inability to accept diagnosis of bone disease and fracture.

Pretest Care

- Explain exam purpose and procedure. Assure patient that test itself is painless. However, some manipulation of body part will be required which may cause temporary discomfort. No preparation is necessary. Make certain that jewelry and metallic objects are removed from area to be radiographed.

Intratest Care

- Encourage patient to follow positional instructions.

Posttest Care

- Evaluate patient outcomes; provide support and counseling.

·············
CLINICAL ALERT

◊ Although orthopedic x-rays can readily be used to diagnose bony disease, general radiography is inadequate to assess condition of cartilage, tendons, or ligaments.
·············

Osmolality

See Kidney Function Tests

Oxygen Saturation (SaO$_2$)

See Arterial Blood Gases (ABGs)

Pancreatic Function Tests   Blood and Urine

Lipase, Amylase and Amylase Excretion/Clearance

These tests are ordered to detect inflammation of the pancreas or salivary glands and to recognize recurrent attacks of acute pancreatitis in persons who exhibit severe abdominal pain.

Indications

- Assess pancreatic and salivary gland function and malfunction.
- Differentiate acute pancreatitis from peptic ulcer and other disorders in which amylase is increased.
- Monitor treatment of pancreatitis.

Expected Test Outcomes

Amylase: 25–130 IU/L (blood)
Amylase excretion clearance urine: Adult: 2–34 U/2 h;
Amylase excretion/clearance blood: Adult: 260–950 Somogyi units/24 h
Lipase: 23–300 U/L.

Test Outcome Deviations

- *Urine amylase increases* in acute pancreatitis, choledocholithiasis, and peptic ulcer.
- *Blood amylase increases* in acute non-hemorrhagic pancreatitis, early in course of disease, and other pancreatic disorders, perforated peptic ulcer, cerebral trauma, salivary gland disease, ruptured tubal pregnancy, and malignant tumors.
- *Blood amylase decreases* in marked destruction of pancreas, severe liver disease, traumas of pregnancy, severe bruises, and severe thyrotoxemia.
- *Lipase increases* in pancreatitis, pancreatic duct and high intestinal obstructions, pancreatic cancer, acute cholecystitis, cirrhosis, and severe renal disease.
- Lipase elevation occurs 24–36 hours after onset of illness and persists for up to 14 days. Lipase may still be high when amylase is back to normal.
- Lipase usually normal with increased amylase in peptic ulcer, mumps, inflammatory bowel disease, and intestinal obstructions.

Interfering Factors

- Drugs that can cause false positives include: salicylates, thiazide diuretics, ACTH, tetracycline, narcotics, large amounts of ethyl alcohol.
- Drugs that can cause false negatives include: glucose, fluorides, oxolates, citrates.
- Newborns and children have very little or no amylase.

Procedure

- A venous blood sample may be collected at the same time a random urine specimen is obtained.
- A 1-hour, 2-hour, or 24-hour timed specimen will be ordered. A 2-hour specimen is usually collected. Collect urine in a clean container; keep refrigerated. See specimen collection guidelines in Chapter 2. Preservation and handling information for 24-hour urine collection is found in Appendix E.

Nursing Role

Use nursing process model following pre-, intra-, and posttest care guidelines in Chapter 1. See page 8 for list of appropriate nursing diagnoses.

Nursing Diagnosis

- Knowledge deficit related to lack or misinterpretation of information provided about purpose and procedure.
- Anxiety and fear related to test outcome and possible need for further treatment.
- Knowledge deficit related to significance of test outcome deviation and related life-style changes.
- High risk for injury related to venipuncture.

Pretest Care

- Assess patient compliance and patient knowledge base prior to explaining test purpose and procedure.

Intratest Care

- Encourage fluids during test if fluids are not restricted for other medical reasons.
- Accurate test results depend upon proper collection, preservation, and labeling. Be sure to include test start and completion times.

Posttest Care

• Evaluate patient outcomes. Provide counseling and support as appropriate.

•••••••••••••

CLINICAL ALERT

◊ The 2-hour amylase excretion in the urine is a more sensitive test than either the serum amylase or lipase test. In patients with acute pancreatitis, the urine often shows a prolonged elevation of amylase as compared to the short-lived peak in the blood.

•••••••••••••

Pap Smear—Papanicolaou Maturation Index (MI), Cytologic Study of Female Genital Tract

Special Study

This test examines cells from vagina, cervix, endocervix, and posterior fornix; is used principally for diagnosis of precancers and cancers of female genital tract.

Indications

• Screen for early detection of cervical cancer.
• Assess hormone cytology (especially in relation to ovarian function) and inflammatory disease.

Expected Test Outcomes

• *Normal:* No abnormal or atypical cells and major cell types.
• *Maturation index* (ratio of parabasal to intermediate to superficial cells):
  Normal child: 80/20/0
  Pregnant (2 months): 0/90/10
  Preovulatory adult: 0/40/60
  Postmenopausal adult (age 60): 65/35/5
  Premenstrual adult: 0/70/30
• *Hormonal effect:* Reported as marked estrogen effect, moderate estrogen effect, slight estrogen effect, atrophic, compatible with pregnancy, and no evaluation (specimens too bloody, inflamed or scanty).
• *Presence of microorganisms:* normal flora, scanty or absent trichomonas, monilia, and mixed bacteria.

Test Outcome Deviations

- Abnormal outcomes based upon 1988 Bethesda System for reporting cervical/vaginal cytological diagnosis; refer to *infection, reactive* and *reparative changes* (inflammation, effects of therapy, radiation, medication, IUDs), *epithelial cell abnormalities*, nonepithelial malignant neoplasms, and *hormone evaluation* (compatible or not with age and history).

Interfering Factors

- Medications (tetracycline, digitalis), use of lubricating vaginal jelly, recent douching, infection, and heavy menstrual flow affect outcomes.

Procedure

- Obtain a specimen from the posterior fornix and external os of the cervix; the sample is spread on slides and placed in preservative or fixative. For hormonal smears, scrape the proximal portion of the lateral vaginal wall, avoiding the cervix; otherwise same as above.
- Label specimen with name, date, age, reason for exam, LMP. and site of specimen, hormone therapy or birth control pills, other meds and any radiation therapy.

Nursing Role

Use nursing process model following pre-, intra-, and posttest care guidelines in Chapter 1. See page 8 for list of appropriate nursing diagnoses.

Nursing Diagnosis

- Knowledge deficit related to lack or misinterpretation of information provided about purpose and procedure.
- Anxiety and embarrassment related to modesty during pelvic exam.

Pretest Care

- Explain purpose and procedure of PAP test. Obtain pertinent history. See procedure for requirements. No douching, vaginal suppositories for 2–3 days prior to test. Empty bladder and rectum prior to exam.

Intratest Care

- Help patient to relax, protect modesty, and provide support.

Posttest Care

- Evaluate patient outcomes and counsel appropriately regarding repeat testing and any need for follow-up biopsies and possible culposcopy. Minimal bleeding may occur within 24 hours in some women. Heavy bleeding is serious and should be reported at once.

Parasites

See Stool Analysis

Parathyroid Hormone Assay—   Blood
Parathyrin, Parathormone
(PTH; PTHN; PTH-C Terminal)

This test measures the parathyroid hormone in the blood—a major factor in calcium metabolism.

Indications

- Diagnose hyperparathyroid disease.
- Distinguish nonparathyroid from parathyroid causes of hypercalcemia, as renal failure or vitamin D deficiency, compensatory responses to hypercalcemia in metastic bone tumors.

Expected Test Outcomes

- Varies greatly with method used—necessary to check with the laboratory regarding test results.
- PTH-N, N-terminal: 236–630 pg/mL as bovine PTH 230–630 ng/L.
- PTH-C, C-terminal: 410–1760 pg/mL as bovine PTH 410–1760 mg/L.
- Parathormone: 20–70 mEq/L.

Test Outcome Deviations

- *Increased parathyroid hormone values*: primary hyperthyroidism, chronic renal failure, pseudohyperparathyroidism (slight increase), vitamin D deficiency (moderate), malabsorption (moderate), rickets (moderate), and osteomalacia (moderate).
- *Decreased parathyroid hormone values*: nonparathyroid hypercalcemia as in vitamins A and D intoxication, magnesium deficiency, Grave's disease, permanent post-operative

hypoparathyroidism (secondary).
- *Increased PTH-N values*: Pseudohypoparathyroidism, secondary hyperparathyroidism, and primary hyperparathyroidism.
- *Decreased PTH-N values*: hypoparathyroidism, neoplasms, and nonparathyroid hypercalcemia.
- *Increased PTH-C values*: pseudohypoparathyroidism, primary hyperparathyroidism, secondary hyperparathyroidism, and neoplasms.
- *Decreased PTH-C values*: hypoparathyroidism and nonparathyroid hypercalcemia.

Interfering Factors
- Recent injection of radioisotopes.
- Elevated blood lipids.
- Milk ingestion may falsely lower levels.
- Thiazide diuretics decrease levels.

Procedure
- 10-hour fasting test—NPO after midnight except water.
- Obtain morning specimen—diurnal rhythm affects PTH levels (check with laboratory if patient normally works night shift).
- 6 mL venous blood (3 mL in two separate vials) is obtained following specimen collection guidelines in Chapter 2. Chill on ice if test not done immediately.
- Obtain a serum calcium level determination at the same time if ordered. The serum PTH and serum calcium levels are important in the differential diagnosis.

Nursing Role
Use nursing process model following pre-, intra-, and posttest care guidelines in Chapter 1. See page 8 for list of appropriate nursing diagnoses.

Nursing Diagnosis
- Knowledge deficit related to lack of information or possible misinterpretation of information provided about procedure, equipment, purpose, and preparation.
- High risk of injury or infection related to venipuncture.

Pretest Care
- Assess patient's knowledge of test.
- Explain purpose and blood test procedure, including fasting for test.

- Assess patient regarding sleep/work patterns, as test outcome is related to diurnal rhythm.

Posttest Care
- Advise patient if results are abnormal and that repeat testing may be necessary.
- Check venipuncture site for bleeding, hematoma, and infection and report immediately to physician.
- Compare parathyroid hormone during test outcome with those of serum calcium levels to aid differential diagnosis.

Partial Pressure of Carbon Dioxide (PCO$_2$)

See Arterial Blood Gases (ABGs)

Partial Pressure of Oxygen (PO$_2$)

See Arterial Blood Gases (ABGs)

Partial Thromboplastin Time (PTT)
Activated Partial Thromboplastin Time (APTT)

See Coagulation Tests

Pelvic Ultrasound

See Gynecologic Sonogram Imaging

pH Blood

See Arterial Blood Gases

PET Scan

See Positron Emission Tomography

Phenylketonuria (PKU)   Blood and Urine

Routine blood and urine tests are done on newborns to detect PKU, a genetic disease characterized by a lack of enzyme that converts phenylalanine to tyrosine that can lead to mental retardation and brain damage if untreated.

Indications

- Neonatal screening test used to detect genetic hepatic enzyme deficiency. May be state mandated.

Expected Test Outcomes

Blood: < 4 mg/100 mL
Urine: Negative dipstick; no observed color change.

Test Outcome Deviations

- In a positive test for PKU, blood phenylalanine is greater than 15 mg/100 mL. Blood tyrosine is less than 5 mg/100 mL. It is never increased in PKU.
- The urine test is positive in PKU.

Interfering Factors

- Premature infants, infants weighing less than 11 kg (5 lb) may have elevated phenylalanine and tyrosine levels without having the genetic disease. This is probably a result of delayed development of appropriate enzyme activity in liver.
- Large amounts of ketones in urine will produce an atypical color reaction.

Procedure (Collecting Blood Sample)

- After skin is cleansed with an antiseptic, infant's heel is punctured with a sterile disposable lancet. If bleeding is slow, it is helpful to hold baby so blood flows with help of gravity. Circles on filter paper must be filled completely. This can best be done by placing one side of the filter paper against infant's heel and watching for blood to appear on front side of the paper and completely fill circle.
- Refer to guidelines for specimen collection in Chapter 2.

Procedure (Collecting Urine Sample)

- The reagent strip is either dipped into a fresh sample of urine or pressed against a wet diaper. Follow manufacturer's directions exactly. Refer to guidelines for specimen collection in Chapter 2.

Nursing Role

Use nursing process model following pre-, intra-, and posttest care guidelines in Chapter 1. See page 8 for list of appropriate nursing diagnoses.

Nursing Diagnosis

• Anxiety of parent related to meaning of test and procedure outcome.
• High risk for injury related to skin puncture.

Pretest Care

• Assess parent knowledge base prior to explaining test purpose and procedure.

Intratest Care

• Accurate test results depend on proper collection, following manufacturer's directions and labeling.

Posttest Care

• Evaluate patient outcome. Provide counseling and support to parent as appropriate.

••••••••••••
CLINICAL ALERTS

◇ The blood test must be performed at least 3 days after birth or after the child has had a chance to ingest protein (milk) for a period of 24–48 hours. Urine testing is done at the 4- or 6-week check-up if a blood sample was not obtained. PKU studies should be done on all infants 5 lb or more before they leave hospital.

••••••••••••

Phosphate (P)

See Electrolyte Studies

Platelet Count

See Complete Blood Count (CBC)

Porphyrins and Porphobilinogens   **Timed Urine**

This test measures porphyrins, cyclic compounds formed from delta-aminolevalinic acid (ALA), important in the formation of hemoglobin and other hemoproteins that function as carriers of oxygen in the blood and tissues.

Indications

- Assess porphyria, liver disease, lead poisoning, and pellegra.

Expected Test Outcomes

Porphobilinogen: 0–2.5 mg/24 h
Porphyrins: 24-hr fractionation µ/24 h

	MALE	FEMALE
Uroporphyrin	8–44	4–22
Coproporphyrin	10–109	3–56
Hepta carboxyporphyrin	0–12	0–9
Penta carboxyporphyrin	0–4	0–3
Hexa carboxyporphyrin	0–5	0–5
Total porphyrin	8–149	3–78

ALA: 0–7.5 mg/24 h

Test Outcome Deviations

- *Increased porphobilinogen* in porphyria; acute intermittent ALA is increased, variegate porphyria, ALA may be normal and hereditary coproporphyrin ALA may be normal.
- *Increased porphyrins;* fractionated acute porphyria ALA is increased, congenital erythropoietic porphyria, hereditary coproporphyrin, and variegate porphyria.
- Chemical porphyria; ALA may be normal, caused by heavy metal poisoning or carbon tetrachloride.
- Lead poisoning; increasedALA in urine; porphobilinogen may be normal
- Other conditions with increased porphyria; viral hepatitis, cirrhosis, and newborn of mother with porphyria.
- Congenital hepatic porphyria ALA may be increased.

Interfering Factors

- Oral contraceptives for susceptible patients.
- Alcohol must be avoided during test.
- Certain drugs interfere with test.

Procedure

- Collect urine in a clean container; refrigeration is usually required. Specimen is kept protected from exposure to light.

See specimen collection guidelines in Chapter 2.
- Standards for 24-hour urine collection and handling are in Appendix E.

Nursing Role

Use nursing process model following pre-, intra-, and posttest care guidelines in Chapter 1. See page 8 for list of appropriate nursing diagnoses.

Nursing Diagnosis
- Knowledge deficit related to lack of information or possible misinterpretation of information provided about procedure, purpose, and preparation.
- Knowledge deficit related to significance of test outcome deviation and related life-style changes.

Pretest Care
- Assess patient compliance.
- Assess patient knowledge base prior to explaining test purpose and procedure.

Intratest Care
- Food and fluids are permitted; alcohol and excessive fluid intake during collection should be avoided.
- Accurate test results depend upon proper collection, preservation, and labeling. Be sure to include test start and completion times.
- Observe and record color of urine. If porphyrins are present, urine may have a grossly recognizable amber-red or burgundy color. It may vary from pale pink to almost black. Some patients will excrete a urine of normal color that turns dark after standing in the light.

Posttest Care
- Evaluate patient outcome. Provide counseling and support as appropriate.

••••••••••••
CLINICAL ALERT
◊ Phenothiazines may cause misleading results. The patient should be off all medications 2–4 weeks prior to testing.
••••••••••••

Positron Emission Tomography (PET)

Nuclear Medicine
Scan Imaging

Positron emission tomography (PET) is the combined use of positron-emitting isotopes and emission-computed axial tomography to measure physiological tissue function.

Indications

- Assess blood flow and tissue metabolism.
- Evaluate epilepsy, dementia, stroke, schizophrenia, and brain tumors.
- Determine cardiac tissue viability, myocardial perfusion, and coronary artery disease.
- Early tumor detecting and staging; monitor therapy.

Expected Test Outcomes

Normal physiological outcomes of body metabolism based on oxygen, glucose, fatty acid utilization, and protein synthesis. Normal blood flow and anatomy are to be visualized.

Test Outcome Deviations

- In *epilepsy* focal areas with increased metabolism have been seen during actual stage of epilepsy, and decreased oxygen utilization and blood flow during interictal stage. In *stroke,* an extremely complex pathophysiologic picture is being revealed: anaerobic glycolysis, depressed oxygen utilization, and decreased blood flow. In *dementia,* decreased glucose consumption (hypometabolic activity) is revealed by PET imaging. Positron emission tomography is used to differentiate Alzheimer's disease and other types of dementia such as Huntington's disease and Parkinson's disease. In *schizophrenia,* some studies using labeled glucose indicate reduced metabolic activity in the frontal region. The PET scans can also distinguish the developmental stages of cranial tumors and give information about operability of such tumors. In *brain tumors,* data have been collected concerning oxygen use and blood flow relationships for these tumors. Gliomas have relatively good perfusion in comparison to their decreased oxygen utilization. The high uptake of radiopharmaceutical in gliomas is reported to correlate with the tumor's histological grade.

- With coronary artery disease, areas of decreased blood flow and/or perfusion occur and indicate myocardial tissue that is no longer viable.
- Abnormal glucose metabolism determines tumor growth. Tumor grading can be assessed by the rate of increases in glucose metabolism. In cases of suspected tumor recurrence after therapy, PET differentiates any new growth from necrotic tissue.

Procedure

- Patient procedures vary and the total time to perform a single scan takes from 1–2 hours. The most commonly used positron-emitting radiopharmaceuticals are nitrogen-13, oxygen-15, and fluoride-18, fluorodoxyglucose (FDG).
- Patient is positioned on a table and positioned within scanner. Prior to administration of radiopharmaceutical, a background transmission scan is performed. In certain procedures, this may be optional.
- The radioactive drug is administered intravenously. Patient must wait 30–45 minutes in department, usually remains on table, and then the area of interest is scanned.

Nursing Role

Use nursing process model following pre-, intra-, and posttest care guidelines in Chapter 1. See page 8 for list of appropriate nursing diagnoses.

Nursing Diagnosis

- Knowledge deficit related to anxiety and lack or misinterpretation of information provided about purpose and procedure.
- High risk of injury (radiation hazard) related to radiopharmaceutical injection.

Pretest Care

- For neurology: advise patient that lying as still as possible during scan is necessary. However, patient is not to fall asleep or count to pass the time.
- Use measures to reduce anxiety and help patient manage stress, such as progressive relaxation and breathing techniques. Excessive anxiety can ruin test results when brain function is being tested.
- For cardiology: an intravenous line may need to be established. Fasting, smoking restrictions, and certain medications

may be required before imaging. Consult with the referring physician and/or the nuclear imaging department.

Intratest Care

- For neurology, it is important to maintain a quiet environment.
- For cardiology, it may be necessary to place ECG leads on patient. See Nuclear Medicine Scan: Overview.

Posttest Care

- Evaluate patient outcomes and counsel appropriately.

2-Hour Postprandial Blood Sugar

See Blood Glucose Tests

Potassium, Blood and Timed Urine

See Electrolyte Studies

Pregnancy Tests— Human Chorionic Gonadotropin (HCG)   Blood and Urine

All pregnancy tests are designed to detect human chorionic gonadotropin (HCG).

Indications

- Confirm pregnancy and estimate gestational age.
- Detect trophoblastic tumors in men.

Expected Test Outcomes

Blood and Urine

Nonpregnant females and men: negative.

Urine

Pregnant female: 1–12 weeks: 6,000–500,000 IU/24 h.
Commercial, over-the-counter pregnancy kits are available. Usually test can be done 3–5 days after missed menstrual period.

Test Outcome Deviations

- *Increased urine* levels usually indicate pregnancy but also present in choriocarcinoma, hydatidiform mole, testicular tumors, chorioepithelioma, chorioadenoma destruens, some ectopic pregnancies, cancer of the lung.
- *Decreased urine* or *negative* levels indicate fetal death, abortion-incomplete or threatened.
- *Increased blood levels* as pregnancy progresses; methadone affects levels.

Interfering Factors

- False negative urine tests and falsely low levels of HCG may be due to a dilute urine (low specific gravity) or a specimen obtained too early in pregnancy.
- False positive urine tests are associated with proteinuria, hematuria, presence of excess pituitary gonadotropin, and certain drugs such as antiparkinsonism drugs, anticonvulsants, hypnotics, phenothiazines.

Procedure

- Serum (1 mL) obtained by venipuncture following specimen colletion guidelines in Chapter 2.
- An early morning specimen is collected in a clean container. This specimen usually contains greatest concentration of HCG. However, specimens collected at any time may be used; but specific gravity must be at least 1.005. See specimen collection guidelines in Chapter 2.
- A 24-hour specimen is collected for quantitative HCG studies. See specimen collection guidelines in Chapter 2.
- General information for 24-hour urine collection are in Appendix E.

Nursing Role

Use nursing process model following pre-, intra-, and posttest care guidelines in Chapter 1. See page 8 for list of appropriate nursing diagnoses.

Nursing Diagnosis

- Knowledge deficit related to lack of or misinterpretation of information provided about purpose and procedure.
- Anxiety and fear related to test outcome and need for further treatment.

Pretest Care

- Assess patient knowledge base prior to explaining test purpose and procedure.
- Ask patient when she had last menstrual period.

Intratest Care

- Accurate test results depend upon proper collection, preservation, and labeling. Be sure to include urine test start, completion, or collection times.
- List any drugs being used on lab slip.
- Grossly bloody specimens are not acceptable; in this instance, a catheterized specimen should be obtained.

Posttest Care

- Evaluate patient outcome. Provide counseling and support as appropriate.

Pregnanediol   Timed Urine

This test measures ovarian and placental function and is indicated when a deficiency of progesterone is suspected.

Indications

- Evaluate amenorrhea and other menstrual disorders.
- Assess placental failure and fetal death.

Expected Test Outcomes

- This test is difficult to standardize; it varies with age, sex, and weeks of pregnancy.
- Excretion high in pregnancy.
- Men: 0–1 mg/24 h
- Women
  Follicular: 0.5–1.5 mg/24 h
  Pregnancy: 6–100 mg/24 h
  Postmenopausal: 0.2–1 mg/24 h
- Child: 0.4–1.0 mg/24 h

Test Outcome Deviations

- *Increased levels* associated with luteal cysts of ovary, arrhenoblastoma of ovary, hyperadrenocorticism, pregnancy, malignant neoplasm of trophoblast.

- *Decreased levels* associated with amenorrhea, threatened abortion, fetal death, toxemia, neoplasm of ovary, ovarian tumor, hydatidiform mole.

Interfering Factors
- Improper specimen collection affects outcome.

Procedure
- Collect urine in a clean container for 24-hour refrigeration; preservative may be required. See timed specimen collection guidelines in Chapter 2 and collection standards in Appendix E.
- Record date of last menstrual period.

Nursing Role
Use nursing process model following pre-, intra-, and posttest care guidelines in Chapter 1. See page 8 for list of appropriate nursing diagnoses.

Nursing Diagnosis
- Knowledge deficit related to lack or misinterpretation of information provided about purpose, procedure, and need for patient cooperation.
- Potential for noncompliance related to need for patient cooperation and timed urine protocols.
- Ineffective individual coping related to test outcome and inability to accept diagnosis, and possible need for further treatment.

Pretest Care
- Assess patient compliance. Obtain accurate menstrual history.
- Assess patient knowledge base prior to explaining test purpose and procedure.

Intratest Care
- Accurate test results depend upon proper collection, preservation, and labeling. Be sure to include test start and completion times.
- Food and fluids are permitted.

Posttest Care
- Evaluate patient outcome. Provide counseling and support as appropriate.

Proctoscopy— Anoscopy, Sigmoidoscopy, Proctosigmoidoscopy

Disorders of the anal canal, rectum, and sigmoid colon linings are visualized, examined, and diagnosed by means of proctosigmoidoscopes, anoscopes or proctoscopes.

Indications

- Routine screening for carcinomas over age 40.
- Evaluate hemorrhoids, blood in the stool, changes in bowel habits, lower abdominal or perineal pain, prolapse.
- Assess anal pruritus or passage of mucus or pus in stool and unexplained anemia.

Expected Test Outcomes

Normal appearing anal canal, rectum, and sigmoid colon mucosa.

Test Outcome Deviations

- Inflammatory processes such as chronic ulcerative colitis, Crohn's disease, acute or chronic proctitis, or pseudomembranous colitis.
- Polyps, ulcers, cysts, bleeding sites, fistulas, strictures, infections, abscesses, stenoses.
- Carcinomas or benign tumors.

Procedure

- Patient is placed in a left lateral position with knees flexed or in a knee-chest position. In left lateral position, buttocks should be over table edge. (Knee-chest position is used with rigid scopes.) Digital examination of anus and rectum is done before endoscopes are carefully inserted and advanced through the anal canal, rectum, and sigmoid colon and then slowly withdrawn. Specimen can be obtained and polyps can be removed during the procedure. Biopsy of anal canal may require an anesthetic be given to patient.
- The actual examination usually takes under 10 minutes.

Nursing Role

Use nursing process model following pre-, intra-, and posttest care guidelines in Chapter 1. See page 8 for list of appropriate nursing diagnoses.

Nursing Diagnosis

• Knowledge deficit related to lack of information or misinterpretation of information provided about purpose and procedure.
• Anxiety related to actual scope procedure.
• Sensory-perceptual alterations related to instrumentation of portions of lower GI tract.
• Body image disturbance related to need for exposure during examination.

Pretest Care

• Explain purpose and procedure of tests. Instruct patient regarding proper dietary restrictions such as light diet evening before and bowel preparation such as enemas or laxatives before the exam.
• Explain that patient may experience gas pains, cramping, and urge to defecate as scope is advanced; slow and deep breathing as well as abdominal muscle relaxation may reduce these sensations. (Sometimes sedatives, tranquilizers, or analgesics may be given prior to the exam.)
• Obtain baseline vital signs.

Intratest Care

• Monitor vital signs per protocols.
• Position patient properly and drape adequately so exposure is minimized.
• Coach patient in performing slow, deep breathing and abdominal muscle relaxation.
• Place specimens in appropriate preservatives, label correctly, and route to lab in a timely manner.

Posttest Care

• Monitor vital signs per protocols.
• Encourage patient to rest for several minutes and to sit up slowly to prevent postural hypotension.
• Be alert to symptoms of a vaso-vagal reaction (hypotension, pallor, diaphoresis, and bradycardia) and notify physician STAT if symptoms occur.
• Explain that large amounts of flatus may be passed because of air in bowel.
• Small amounts of blood in the stool may be expected if biopsy or polypectomy was done. Instruct patient to watch for

signs of bowel perforation and to contact physician immediately if perforation is suspected (see Clinical Alerts).

....
CLINICAL ALERT

◊ Men over age 45 are at higher risk for adenocarcinoma of the rectum.

◊ Symptoms of bowel perforation (an infrequent event) include rectal bleeding or hemorrhage, abdominal distention and pain, fever, and malaise. The physician needs to be notified STAT.

◊ Patients presenting acute signs and symptoms or pregnant women should not be given bowel preps unless specifically ordered by the physician.

....

Progesterone   Blood

The test is done to confirm ovulation and evaluate function of corpus luteum.

Indications

• Study fertility.
• Assess ovarian production of progesterone.

Expected Test Outcomes

	NG/ML
Male	0–0.4
Female	
follicular	0.1–1.5
luteal	2.5–28.1
1st trimester	9–47
2nd trimester	16.8–146
3rd trimester	55–255
>60	0–0.2
prepubertal	0.1–0.3
midluteal	5.7–28.1
oral contraceptives	0.1–0.3

Test Outcome Deviations

• *Increases* in congenital adrenal hyperplasia, lipid ovarian tumor, molar pregnancy, and chorionepithelioma of ovary.

- *Decreases* in threatened abortion and galactorrhea-amenorrhea syndrome.

Procedure

- Serum (5–7 mL) obtained by venipuncture according to specimen collection guidelines in Chapter 2.
- Note sex, age, day of LMP, and trimester of pregnancy on lab slip or computer screen.

Nursing Role

Use nursing process model following pre-, intra-, and posttest care guidelines in Chapter 1. See page 8 for list of appropriate nursing diagnoses.

Nursing Diagnosis

- Knowledge deficit related to lack or misinterpretation of information provided about purpose and procedure.
- Anxiety related to test outcomes and diagnosis of infertility and ovarian dysfunction.
- High risk for injury related to venipuncture.

Pretest Care

- Explain purpose and procedure.

Posttest Care

- Evaluate patient outcomes and counsel appropriately.

Prolactin (HPRL)   Blood

This test measures the amount of this pituitary hormone (essential for initiating and maintaining lactation), in presence of amenorrhea, milky discharge from breasts, and infertility.

Indications

- Diagnose and manage prolactin-secreting pituitary tumors.
- Evaluate galactorrhea and amenorrhea.
- In males, evaluate impotence, gynecomastia, and hypogonadism.

Expected Test Outcomes

Nonpregnant women: 0–17 ng/mL
Pregnant women: < 400 ng/mL or µg/L by third trimester
Men: < 15 ng or µg/L.

Test Outcome Deviations

- Increase in galactorrhea, amenorrhea, prolactin-secreting pituitary tumors, infertility, ectopic malignant tumors, hypothyroidism, renal failure, and anorexia nervosa.

Interfering Factors

- Many drugs may increase (estrogens, antidepressants, antihypertensives) or decrease values.
- Increase in newborns, pregnancy, postpartum, stress, exercise, drugs, nipple stimulantion, and lactation.

···············
CLINICAL ALERT

◊ Normal prolactin level does not rule out pituitary tumor.
···············

Procedure

- A 12-hour fasting (5 mL) serum obtained by venipuncture according to specimen collection guidelines in Chapter 1. Draw specimen between 5–10 AM.

Nursing Role

Use nursing process model following pre-, intra-, and posttest care guidelines in Chapter 1. See page 8 for list of appropriate nursing diagnoses.

Nursing Diagnosis

- Knowledge deficit related to lack or misinterpretation of information provided about purpose and procedure.
- Anxiety related to test outcomes and relationship to fertility.
- High risk for injury related to venipuncture.

Pretest Care

- Explain purpose, procedure, and fasting.

Posttest Care

- Evaluate patient outcome and counsel appropriately.

Prostate-Specific Antigen (PSA)

See Tumor Markers

————

Prostate Ultrasound—   Ultrasound Imaging
Prostate Sonography,
Transrectal Sonography
of the Prostate

This noninvasive procedure images the prostate and surrounding tissues.

Indications

- Evaluate an abnormality detected on digital exam or by deviations in serum levels of prostate-specific antigen (PSA).
- Staging of biopsy-proven prostate carcinoma.
- Evaluate infertility related to prostate pathology.
- Guidance for biopsy or other interventional procedures.

Expected Test Outcomes

Normal size and consistency of prostate gland.

Test Outcome Deviations

- Prostate enlargement (glandular hypertrophy), presence of space-occupying lesions: tumors, abscesses, cysts, and prostatitis.

Interfering Factors

- Fecal material in rectum will obscure visualization of prostate.

Procedure

- Patient is asked to lie on an exam table on his left side with knees bent toward chest.
- A draped and lubricated rectal transducer is inserted into rectum. Water may be introduced to sheath surrounding transducer head. Patient may feel slight pressure. Transducer handle is rotated in order to produce images in a variety of planes.
- Total exam time is approximately 15–30 minutes.

Nursing Role

Use nursing process model following pre-, intra-, and posttest care guidelines in Chapter 1. See page 8 for list of appropriate nursing diagnoses.

Nursing Diagnosis

- Knowledge deficit related to lack of information or possible misinterpretation of information provided about procedure, purpose, and preparation.
- Anxiety and fear related to perception of diagnostic procedure as frightening or embarrassing.
- Powerlessness related to unfamiliar procedure, equipment.
- Ineffective coping related to test outcome and inability to accept diagnosis of prostate disease.
- Decisional conflict related to test outcome and potential for interventional procedures.

Pretest Care

- Explain purpose and procedure. Assure patient that no radiation is employed and that test is painless.
- Instruct patient to administer a cleansing enema 1 hour prior to exam to eliminate fecal material from rectum.

Posttest Care

- Evaluate patient outcomes; provide support and counselling.

··············
CLINICAL ALERT

◇ Patient must agree to sign a surgical permit prior to performance of ultrasound-guided biopsy or other interventional procedures. See Ultrasound: Overview.
··············

Protein   Blood and Urine

Total Protein, Protein Electrophoresis (PE), Serum Protein Electrophoresis (SPE), Albumins, Globulins, Albumin Globulin Ratio (A/G), Alpha 1 and 2 Globulins, Gamma Globulin

These measurements and the correlates of specific protein pattern changes are helpful in identifying various disease states such as dysprotenemia, hypogammoglobulinemias, and some inflammatory and neoplastic states.

Indications

- Screening test, not definitive for a particular disorder.
- Index of nutrition and osmotic pressure in edematous and malnourished patient.

- Assess immune function.
- Aids diagnosis of multiple myeloma, Waldenstrom's macroglobulinemia, hypogammaglobunemia, afibrinogenemia, atransferrinemia.

Expected Test Outcomes

Total protein: Adult	6.0–8.6 g/dL
Albumin: Adult	3.8–5.6 g/dL
Globulin	2.3–3.5 g/dL
A/G Radio	1.0–2.2
Alpha-1-globulin	0.1–0.3 g/dL
Alpha-2-globulin	0.6–1.0 g/dL
Beta-globulin	0.7–1.4 g/dL
Gamma-globulin	0.7–1.6 g/dL

Globulin
  <5 d: 5.4–7.0 g/dL
  1–3 y: 5.9–7.0 g/dL
  4–6 y: 5.5–7.8 g/dL
  7–9 y: 6.2–8.1 g/dL
  10–19 y: 6.3–8.6 g/dL

Albumin
  <5 d: 2.6–3.6 g/dL
  1–3 y: 3.4–4.2 g/dL
  4–6 y: 3.5–5.2 g/dL
  7–9 y: 3.7–5.6 g/dL
  10–19 y: 3.7–5.6 g/dL

Test Outcome Deviations

- *Total protein increases* (hyperproteinemia) due to hemoconcentration as result of dehydration with body fluid losses and poor kidney function.
- *Total protein decreases* (hypoproteinemia) in starvation, malabsorption, severe hemorrhage, liver disease, alcoholism, chronic glomerulonephritis, diarrhea, severe dermatitis and burns; heart failure, hyperthyroidism, and prolonged immobilization.
- *Albumin increases* generally not found except in dehydration.
- *Albumin decreases* in multiple myeloma and Hodgkin's, lymphatic leukemia, nephrosis and nephritis, peptic ulcer and ulcerative colitis, malnutrition, essential hypertension and congestive heart failure, stress and burns, collagen diseases, hyperthyroidism, diabetes.

- *Alpha-1-globulin increases* in Hodgkin's, metastic carcinomas, protein losing enteropathy, and stress.
- *Alpha-1 decreases* with juvenile pulmonary emphysema.
- *Alpha-2 increases* in Hodgkin's, chronic glomerulonephritis, stress, acute inflammatory and infectious disease, collagen diseases, and diabetes.
- *Alpha-2 decreases* in Laennec's cirrhosis and acute viral hepatitis.
- *Increased beta globulin* in analbuminemia, rheumatoid arthritis, and diabetes.
- *Decreased beta globulin* in lymphatic leukemia, lymphoma, monocytic and mychogenous leukemia, ulcerative colitis, acute viral hepatitis, and disseminated intravascular coagulation (DIC).
- *Increased gamma globulin* in multiple myeloma, macroglobulinemia, myelogross and monocytic leukemias, analbuminemia, hypersensitivity, and acute viral hepatitis.
- *Decreased gammaglobulin* in lymphatic leukemia, hypogammaglobulinemia, and protein losing enteropathies.
- Rarely are there increases or decreases in the beta globulins without the alteration being related to some disorder in the gamma globulin function.

Interfering Factors

- Gross hemolysis affects test outcome.
- Fibrinogen (if plasma collected instead of serum) can migrate between beta and gamma regions causing "bridging" effect. If a new serum sample is unobtainable, the sample can be treated with thrombin to remove the fibrinogen.
- Many drugs affect test patterns, especially salicylates, steroids, and antibiotics, also excessive IVs.
- Decreased total protein and albumin in pregnancy; supine position causes decreases.

Procedure

- Serum (10 mL) obtained by venipuncture according to specimen collection guidelines in Chapter 2. Assure that blood sample is not collected in an anticoagulant as serum, not plasma, is required.
- If it is possible for a 24-hour urine to be collected, make appropriate arrangements as it is preferable to a random urine sample.
- Submit 25 mL from a 24-hour urine collection, if a urine protein electrophoresis is to be run simultaneously.

- Urine protein electrophoresis is used primarily to identify Bence Jones protein. If required, follow 24-hour urine specimen collection guidelines in Chapter 2.
- Indicate drugs that may affect outcome on lab slip or computer screen.
- See Appendix E for standards of timed urine collection.

Nursing Role

Use nursing process model following pre-, intra-, and posttest care guidelines in Chapter 1. See page 8 for list of appropriate nursing diagnoses.

Nursing Diagnosis

- Knowledge deficit related to lack of or possible misinterpretation of information provided about blood and/or urine procedure and purpose and need for patient cooperation.
- High risk for injury or infection related to venipuncture.
- Knowledge deficit related to abnormal test outcomes and need for repeat testing.

Pretest Care

- Assess patient's understanding of tests for immune function; provide information about a lymphoproliferative disorder should the SPE be abnormal. Acute and/or chronic inflammation and infection can also be represented by an abnormal SPE pattern. Advise the patient that further testing may be necessary.

Posttest Care

- Evaluate patient outcomes, monitor, and counsel appropriately. Very low protein < 4 gm/dL and low albumin can cause edema. Observe, report, and document signs and symptoms of possible accompanying edema.
- Follow-up with collecting appropriate sample for Immunofixation Electrophoresis (see Immune Function Tests) the SPE demonstrates the type of the serum proteins and the pathologist's interpretation recommend further testing.

Protein   Timed Urine

This test measures the amount of protein in the urine. The persistent presence of protein in urine is the single most important indication of renal disease.

Indications

- Indication of severity of renal disease.
- Differential diagnosis of renal disease.

Expected Test Outcomes

Adult: 10–140 mg/L in 24 h or 1–14 mg/dL.
Child (< 10): 10–100 mg/L in 24 h or 1–10 mg/dL.

Test Outcome Deviations

- Increased levels occur in renal diseases such as nephritis, glomerulonephritis, nephrosis, renal vein thrombosis, malignant hypertension, SLE, and pyelonephritis.
- May occur in following non-renal diseases and conditions such as fever, acute infections, traumas, severe anemias and leukemia, toxemias, diabetes, vascular disease; and poisoning from turpentine, phosphorus, mercury, sulfosalicylic acid, lead, phenol, opiates, and drug therapy; myeloma, and Waldemstrom's macroglobulinemia.

Interfering Factors

- Strenuous exercise, severe emotional stress, and cold baths.
- Drugs can cause false negatives and false positives (cephalo--sporins, sulfonamides, penicillin, gentamicin, tolbutamide, acetazolamide, and contrast media).
- Alkaline urine can give false positive results.
- Very dilute urine can give falsely low protein value.
- False or accidental proteinuria may be present because of a mixture of pus and red blood cells in urinary tract infections and the menstrual flow.
- Increased protein occurs after eating large amounts of protein, pregnancy, newborn infants, in premenstrual state.

Procedure

- Collect urine in a clean container and test as soon as possible. See specimen collection guidelines in Chapter 2. General information for 24 hour urine collection are in Appendix E.

Nursing Role

Use nursing process model following pre-, intra-, and posttest care guidelines in Chapter 1. See page 8 for list of appropriate nursing diagnoses.

Nursing Diagnosis

- Knowledge deficit related to lack of information or possible misinterpretation of information provided about procedure and purpose.
- Potential for noncompliance to test protocols related to confusion, weakness, and other individual factors.
- Impaired adjustment related to acceptance of test outcome and kidney disease.

Pretest Care

- Assess patient compliance.
- Assess patient knowledge base prior to explaining test purpose and procedure.

Intratest Care

- The same amount of liquids should be consumed during the collection period as is normally consumed unless otherwise instructed.
- Accurate test results depend upon proper collection, preservation, and labeling. Be sure to include test start and completion times.

Posttest Care

- Evaluate patient outcome. Provide counseling and support as appropriate.

. . . .
CLINICAL ALERT

◊ >2000 mg/day or >40 mg/day in children; usually indicates glomerular etiology.

◊ >3500 mg/day points to a nephrotic syndrome.
. . . .

Protein Electrophoresis

See Protein Blood and Urine

Prothrombin Time, Pro-Time (PT)

See Coagulation Studies

Pulmonary Function Tests (PFTs), Spirometry

Special Study

Airflow, Lung Volume, Gas Diffusion,
FVC, FEV, FEF, PIFR, VC, IC

Pulmonary function tests (PFTs) are used to evaluate the nature and extent of pulmonary disease and to identify the underlying ventilatory impairment as obstructive and/or restrictive.

Indications

- *Air flow (rates)* quantify the degree of airway obstruction and assess responses to inhaled bronchodilators and/or bronchial provocations.
- *Lung volume (physiologic air-containing compartments—not anatomical)* determines if there is air trapping or hyperventilation of the lung and differentiate an obstructive vs. a restrictive ventilatory impairment.
- *Diffusion capacity (gas transfer rate across alveolar capular membrane)* determines whether or not a gas exchange defect exists. Although gas exchange problems are generally associated with ventilatory impairments, there are cases in which the diffusion capacity may be affected without coexisting lung disease, eg, anemia.
- Monitor for pulmonary side effects of such drugs as bleomycin, which can cause interstitial pneumonitis or fibrosis.

Expected Test Outcomes

Air Flow Rates—Volume-Time Tracing

- Forced vital capacity (FVC) = maximum amount of air exhaled during the maneuver, expressed in liters; should be > 80% of predicted value.
- Forced expiratory volume in one second (FEV1.0) = amount of air exhaled in first second of FVC, expressed in liters; should be >80% of predicted value.
- FEV1.0/FVC = ratio of amount of air exhaled in first second as compared to total, expressed as a percent; should be > 70%.
- Forced Expiratory Flow during middle 50% (FEF25–75) = average flow of air during middle 50% of the FVC, expressed in liters per second; should be 50% of predicted value.

Flow Volume Loop

- Peak expiratory flow rate (PEFR) = maximum flow attained during forced expiratory maneuver, expressed in liters per second or per minute.
- Forced expiratory flow at 25, 50, and 75% (FEF25, FEF50 and FEF75) = instantaneous airway flow rates at 25, 50 and 75% of patient's lung volume respectively, expressed in liters per second.
- Peak inspiratory flow rate (PIFR) = maximum flow attained during forced inspiratory maneuver, expressed in liters per second.

•••••••••••••

CLINICAL ALERT

◊ If the spirometry test is used to assess response to inhaled bronchodilators, an increase in FEV1 of at least 10–12% is considered significant. When using spirometry to determine presence or absence of bronchial hyperreactivity, a decrease in FEV1 of >20% is considered positive.

•••••••••••••

Lung Volumes

Part I Test

- Vital capacity (VC) = maximum amount of air exhaled slowly from a maximum inspiration expressed in liters; should be >80% of predicted value.
- Inspiratory capacity (IC) = maximum amount of air inspired from resting expiratory level expressed in liters; the IC is approximately 75% of VC.
- Expiratory reserve volume (ERV) = maximum amount of air expired from resting expiratory level expressed in liters; ERV is approximately 25% of VC.

Part II Test

- Functional residual capacity (FRC) = amount of air left in lungs at resting expiratory level expressed in liters; 75%–125% of predicted value.
- Residual volume (RV) = amount of air left in lungs at maximal expiration expressed in liters; 75%–125% of predicted value.
- Total lung capacity (TLC) = amount of air contained within lungs at maximum inspiration expressed in liters; should be > 80% of predicted value.

- RV/TLC = ratio of residual volume to total lung capacity expressed as a percentage; normal range is 20–35%.

Diffusion Capacities

- The diffusion capacity of the lung for carbon monoxide (DLCO) = rate of gas transfer (CO) across the alveolar-capillary membrane expressed as mL of CO/min/mmHg; should be > 80% of the predicted value.
- The DLCO per unit of lung volume (DLCO/VL or DLCO/VA) = rate of diffusion per liter of lung volume expressed in mL/min/mmHg per L; should be > 80% of predicted value.
- The diffusion capacity of the lung for oxygen (DLO$_2$) = rate of oxygen exchange across alveolar-capillary membrane expressed as mL of O$_2$/min/mm Hg and is estimated from the DLCO by multiplying DLCO by 1.23.

Test Outcome Deviations: Air Flow Rates

- *Decreases in rates* (eg, FEV1, FEF25–75) consistent with an obstructive ventilatory impairment, typically seen in asthma, chronic bronchitis, and emphysema.
- *Decrease in volume* of air exhaled (FVC) consistent with a restrictive ventilatory impairment seen in interstitial pulmonary fibrosis, obesity, sarcoidosis, and thoracic cage deformities.

Test Outcome Deviations: Lung Volumes

- *Disproportionate increases in the FRC and RV* consistent with air-trapping or overdistention and commonly seen in obstructive ventilatory impairments, as asthma, emphysema, and cystic fibrosis.
- *Decreases in FRC, RV, and TLC* demonstrate reduced lung volume consistent with restrictive ventilatory impairments, as pulmonary interstitial fibrosis, lung restriction, obesity, and asbestosis.

Diffusion Capacity

- *Reductions in DLCO* consistent with gas exchange defects when there is loss of diffusing membrane as in obstructive diseases (emphysema) and restrictive diseases (pulmonary fibrosis), anemia, and space-occupying lesions.

Interfering Factors

- Inhaled bronchodilators, caffeine intake, and smoking may affect results.
- As the spirometry test is patient effort dependent, any acute illness, nausea, GI disturbance, migraine headache, abdominal or chest pain, and recent respiratory infection may affect the results. Also, inability to hold breath or anything that will not permit an airtight seal, as nasogastric tubes, tracheal stoma, perforated eardrum, and if a patient is on continuous oxygen and cannot be taken off for a few minutes.
- Elevated carboxyhemoglobin levels, seen in smokers, can cause a decrease in the DLCO due to the "back pressure" of carbon monoxide.

Procedures

- Patient's demographic data (e.g., age, height, weight, sex, and race) are recorded and via regression equations, the predicted values are determined.

Air Flow Rate Procedure

- In a seated or standing position, with a noseclip on, patient is instructed to inhale maximally and then exhale forcibly, rapidly, and completely into a mouthpiece. The mouthpiece is connected to a *spirometer* via a breathing tube and a recording of the forced expiration is made.
- A minimum of 3 forced expiratory maneuvers are performed with an appropriate rest period between each effort. The two best spirograms should compare within ±5% or 100 mL, whichever is greater, or additional forced maneuvers (practical upper limit of 8) will be required. The best test results, corrected to body temperature pressure saturated (BTPS), are reported and compared with the predicted values determined in step 1.

Lung Volume Procedure

- This is a two-part test which consists of measurement of the vital capacity and the functional residual capacity and their subdivisions.
- Part I—The vital capacity (VC) maneuver is performed on a spirometer by having patient in a seated position, with noseclips on, breathing normally, inspire maximally, and then exhale slowly and fully. From the resultant tracing, the VC and its subdivisions are determined.

• Part II—The functional residual capacity (FRC) is commonly measured either by the helium dilution closed-circuit technique or the nitrogen washout open-technique. The helium dilution technique requires patient to breathe a low concentration of helium (approximately 10%) for several minutes. The volume and concentration of helium are measured before and after the test. The nitrogen washout technique requires the patient to breathe 100% oxygen for several minutes during which the volume and nitrogen concentration of the exhaled air is measured. The FRC is determined from either technique by simple algebraic substitution and the appropriate corrections. With either method, the patient is seated, with a noseclip on, and breathes into a mouthpiece connected to a spirometer and other requisite instrumentation.

• Both procedures are repeated at least twice and the volumes and capacities should compare within ±5% The best test results (in some cases the average), corrected to body temperature pressure saturated (BTPS), are reported and compared against the predicted values determined in Step 1.

Diffusion Capacity Procedure

• Patient's demographic data (e.g., age, height, weight, sex, and race) are recorded and via regression equations the predicted values determined.

• In seated position, with noseclip attached, patient is instructed to exhale maximally and then inspire maximally a diffusion gas mixture (10% helium, 0.3% carbon monoxide, balance room air) through a mouthpiece attached to the pulmonary function analyzer. Following a 10–15 second breathhold, patient is instructed to exhale and a sample of alveolar gas captured for analysis.

• The procedure is repeated and the second diffusion capacity measurement should compare within ±10% or 3 mL of CO/min/mm Hg, whichever is greater. The average result, corrected to standard temperature pressure dry (STPD), is reported and compared against predicted values determined in Step 1. Also, corrections for anemia, altitude, and carboxyhemoglobin are recommended.

Nursing Role

Use nursing process model following pre-, intra-, and posttest care guidelines in Chapter 1. See page 8 for list of appropriate nursing diagnoses.

Nursing Diagnosis

- Knowledge deficit related to lack or misinterpretation of information provided about purpose, procedure, equipment, and need for patient cooperation.
- Anxiety related to testing procedure and patient ability to complete procedure because of known breathing difficulties.

Pretest Care

- Assess for interfering factors and contraindications to testing, such as pain with old bronchodilators for 6–8 h, if tolerated..
- Explain purpose and procedure, emphasizing that this is a noninvasive test requiring cooperation and effort. Combined tests take approximately 20–30 minutes. Patient should be encouraged not to smoke and to go ahead and eat if test is scheduled near meal time.

Intratest Care

- Patient may experience lightheadedness, shortness of breath, and/or slight chest discomfort. These symptoms are transitory and an appropriate rest period between maneuvers is generally all that is needed. Should symptoms persist, technologist will terminate testing and report the data at that time. Although it is a rare event, momentary loss of consciousness, due to anoxia during the forced expiration, has been reported.

Posttest Care

- Assess complaints of slight fatigue and/or chest discomfort related to use of respiratory muscles during deep inspirations followed by forced expirations. This is an expected outcome. Provide for rest as necessary.
- Evaluate other patient outcomes and counsel appropriately.

Radioactive Iodine (RA) Uptake Test

Nuclear Medicine
Scan Imaging

This direct test of the function of the thyroid gland measures ability of the gland to concentrate and retain radioactive iodine.

Indications

- Evaluate hyperthyroid and hypothyroid conditions and assist in staging thyroiditis.
- Check thyroid response to medication for pituitary or hypo-

thalamic dysfunction and effectiveness of radioiodine therapy.
- Part of a complete thyroid workup for symptomatic patients (swollen neck, neck pain, jittery or sluggish).

Expected Test Outcomes

Values are laboratory dependent:
- 1%–13% absorbed by thyroid gland after 2 hours
- 5%–20% absorbed by thyroid gland after 6 hours
- 15%–40% absorbed by thyroid gland after 24 hours

Test Outcome Deviations

- *Increased uptake* (e.g., 20% in 1 hour, 25% in 6 hours, 45% in 24 hours) suggests hyperthyroidism.
- *Decreased uptake* (e.g., 0% in 2 hours, 3% in 6 hours, 10% in 24 hours) may be caused by hypothyroidism.
- NOTE: Decreased uptake is observed in patients with rapid diuresis, renal failure, malabsorption.

Interfering Factors

- Many chemicals, drugs and foods interfere by *lowering uptake* such as iodized foods and iodine-containing drugs, x-ray contrast media used in IVP and CAT scans, (1 week to 1 year or more in duration), antithyroid drugs such as propylthiouracil and related compounds (2–10 days' duration), and thyroid medications such as cytomel, desiccated thyroid, thyroxine synthroid (1–2 weeks' duration), and many others including sulfonamides, orinase, corticosteroids, PAS, isoniazid, phenylbutazone (Butazolidin), antihistamines, ACTH, aminosalicylic acid, and anticoagulants.
- Many drugs and conditions interfere by *enhancing uptake* such as pregnancy, cirrhosis and renal failure, barbiturates, lithium carbonate, phenothiazines (1 week), and iodine deficient diets.

Procedure

- Test is usually done in conjunction with a thyroid scan and assessment of thyroid hormone levels. A fasting state is preferred. A good history and listing of all medications is a must for this test.
- A liquid form or a tasteless capsule of radioiodine is administered orally. (Can be administered intravenously if a quick test is desired.) The patient is usually instructed not to eat for 1 hour after administration of radioiodine.

- Two, six, and 24 hours later, the amount of radioactivity is measured in the thyroid gland. There is no pain or discomfort involved.
- The patient will have to return to the laboratory at the designated time; for the exact time of measurement is crucial in determining uptake.

Nursing Role

Use nursing process model following pre-, intra-, and posttest care guidelines in Chapter 1. See page 8 for list of appropriate nursing diagnoses.

Nursing Diagnosis

- Knowledge deficit related to lack of or misinterpretation of information provided about purpose and procedure.
- High risk for injury/radiation hazard related to administration of radiopharmaceutical.
- Potential for noncompliance related to patient/procedure requirements.

Pretest Care

- Explain purpose, procedure, fasting and scan times. Reassure regarding safety of radiopharmaceutical. Record accurate weight.
- Advise that iodine intake is restricted for at least 1 week before testing and stress compliance with various procedural steps.
- Assess for iodine allergy and consult with physician regarding these data.

•••••••••••••
CLINICAL ALERT

◊ This test is contraindicated in pregnant or lactating women, in children, and in infants.
- Schedule this test before any other radionuclide procedures are done, before any iodine medications are given, and before any x-rays using iodine contrast are done.
◊ See Nuclear Medicine Scans: Overview.
•••••••••••••

Intratest Care

- Stress compliance. Reassure that test is proceeding normally. Provide support.

Posttest Care

- Evaluate patient outcomes and counsel appropriately.
- Pregnant staff and visitors are to avoid prolonged contact for 24–48 hours after radioactive administration.
- Document any problems that may have occurred with the patient during the procedure.
- Body fluids and excretions can undergo routine disposal procedures unless patient is also receiving in vivo radiation therapy.

Radioallergosorbent Test   Blood
(RAST)—Allergens-IgE Antibodies

This test measures the increase and quantity of allergen-specific immunoglobulin-E (IgE) antibodies and is done to identify allergens to which patient has an immediate hypersensitivity.

Indications

- Identify specific allergens that cause asthma, hay fever, atopic eczema, other rashes, and drug reactions.
- Monitor response of patient to therapy.
- Accurate and convenient substitute for skin testing, easier to perform, less painful and less dangerous to patient than skin testing. Useful when skin tests are negative, but clinical history suggests IgE antibodies hypersensitivity, and when a skin disorder prevents accurate reading of skin test.

Expected Test Outcomes

- Test results are reported as a negative or positive as compared with a reference serum tested simultaneously.

Test Outcome Deviations

- Detection of an allergen-specific IgE indicates immediate hypersensitivity to an allergen. A positive RAST is diagnostic of allergy to a particular allergen or allergens, irrespective of the level of total IgE. A positive test is more than 400% of the control.

Interfering Factors

- A radioactive scan within 1 week before sample collection may affect accuracy of test results, because radioimmunoassay is done in laboratory to obtain results.

- Preparation of reliable allergens for use in laboratory testing may cause problems, such as difficulties encountered in recognition and purification of specific allergens.

Procedure

- Serum (4–10 mL) for each group of six RAST tests obtained by venipuncture according to specimen collection guidelines in Chapter 2.

Nursing Role

Use nursing process model following pre-, intra-, and posttest care guidelines in Chapter 1. See page 8 for list of appropriate nursing diagnoses.

Nursing Diagnosis

- Knowledge deficit related to lack of information or possible misinterpretation of information provided about procedure and purpose.
- High risk for injury and/or infection related to venipuncture.
- Knowledge deficit related to positive RAST and need for medical therapy or possible life-style alterations to avoid specific allergens.

Pretest Care

- Assess patient's knowledge of test, medication use, dietary history, and environmental situation in relation to potential allergens.
- Explain purpose and blood test procedure. No fasting is required. Explain that the serum is first screened with a selected panel of six allergens and then followed, if appropriate, by an extended panel of additional allergens.

Posttest Care

- Advise the patient if the test is positive (elevated serum IgE levels) to the specific allergen(s).
- Since additional allergen may be continually added from more than 100 such categories as grasses, trees, molds, weeds, animal danders, foods, and house dust, failure to identify the allergy by the six allergens in the RAST panel may result in further specific testing.
- Once allergen is identified, teach patient what to avoid, such as specific medications, foods, animals, dust, and other allergens.

- If medication therapy is begun, instruct patient regarding therapy program.

Red Blood Cell Count (RBC)

See Complete Blood Count (CBC)

Renal Ultrasound

See Kidney Sonogram

Renogram— Renal Kidney Scan

Nuclear Medicine Scan Imaging Blood and Urine

This nuclear scan studies kidney function, detects renal parenchymal or vascular disease, excretion defects, and permits visualization of renal clearance.

Indications

- Detect unilateral kidney disease and obstruction in upper urinary tract.
- Study hypertensive patient for renal cause.
- When urethral catheterization and IVP is contraindicated or impossible.
- Assess renal transplants.

Expected Test Outcomes

- Normal and equal blood flow in both kidneys.

Test Outcome Deviations

- Diminished blood supply, decreased renal function, renal failure, and renal transplant rejection. Hypertension and obstruction due to stones or traumas.

Interfering Factors

- Antihypertensive medications.

Procedure

- The patient is usually placed in an upright position in front of the camera. Imaging with camera starts immediately upon injection.

- The radiopharmaceutical (technetium) is injected intravenously. An intravenous diuretic may also be administered.
- Imaging with the camera is started immediately upon injection.
- A urine sample or a blood specimen may be obtained at the end of the procedure. Bladder catheterization is necessary in persons with suspected distal ureteral obstruction. See collection guidelines in Chapter 2.

Nursing Role

Use nursing process model following pre-, intra-, and posttest care guidelines in Chapter 1. See page 8 for list of appropriate nursing diagnoses.

Nursing Diagnosis

- Knowledge deficit related to lack or misinterpretation of information provided about purpose, procedure, and radiopharmaceutical.
- Fear and mistrust related to nuclear medicine scan procedures.
- High risk for injury/radioactive hazard related to high dose of radiopharmaceutical injection for renal scan.
- Risk for infection at IV injection site.

Pretest Care

- Record accurate weight. Explain purpose, procedure, and that it will take about 30 minutes. Reassure regarding safety of injection of radiopharmaceutical. See alphabetical list for Nuclear Scans: Overview.
- Before testing, patient should eat and be well hydrated (unless contraindicated).

Intratest Care

- Provide reassurance and support.

Posttest Care

- Encourage fluids and frequent bladder emptying to promote excretion of radionuclide.
- Evaluate patient outcomes, counsel, and monitor appropriately. Assess IV site for signs of infection.
- Dispose of body fluids and excretions following routine procedures unless patient is also receiving therapeutic radiopharmaceuticals to treat disease.

• Pregnant staff and visitors are to avoid prolonged contact with patient for 24–48 hours after radioactive administration.

Reticulocyte Count   Blood

This test measures immature red blood cells and is done in the differential diagnosis of anemia.

Indications

• Differentiate anemias due to bone marrow failure from those due to hemorrhage or red cell destruction.
• Monitor effectiveness of treatment and recovery of bone marrow function.
• Determine radiation effects.

Expected Test Outcomes

Men: 0.5%–1.5% or 0.005–0.015
Women: 0.5%–2.5% or 0.005–0.025
Infants: 2%–5% or 0.020–0.050
Children: 0.5%–4% or 0.005–0.0040
Absolute reticulocyte count = % reticulocytes × erythrocyte count
Reticulocyte index = 1.0

AGE	$\times 10^3$
0–2 wk	82.0–366.0
2–4 wk	80.0–360.0
4–8 wk	20.0–90.0
2–6 mo	19.0–84.0
6 mo–1 y	19.0–78.0
1–6 y	19.5–79.5
6–16 y	20.0–78.0
16–18 y	21.0–81.0
≥ 18 y, male	22.5–82.5
≥ 18 y, female	20.0–75.0

Test Outcome Deviations

• *Reticulocytes increase* in hemolytic anemias, hemoglobinopathies, sickle cell anemias, 3–4 days after hemorrhage, increased RBC destruction, and treatment of anemias.
• *Reticulocytes decrease* in iron deficiency and aplastic anemia, untreated pernicious anemia, chronic infection, radiation

therapy and exposure, marrow tumors, endocrine disorders, and myelodysplastic syndromes.

Procedure

- A small blood sample is obtained by venipuncture according to collection guidelines in Chapter 2.
- A blood smear is prepared and examined microscopically.

Nursing Role

Use nursing process model following pre-, intra-, and posttest care guidelines in Chapter 1. See page 8 for list of appropriate nursing diagnoses.

Nursing Diagnosis

- Knowledge deficit related to lack of or misinterpretation of information provided about purpose and procedure.
- High risk for injury and infection related to venipuncture.

Pretest Care

- Explain purpose and procedure of testing. No fasting is required.

Posttest Care

- Evaluate patient outcome and counsel regarding possible repeat testing and iron medications.
- Plan care based upon test outcomes that reveal anemias and associated weaknesses.

Retrograde Pyelogram   X-Ray Imaging
                          with Contrast

This x-ray examination of the upper urinary tract involves the introduction of a catheter into the ureter(s) through a cystoscope to visualize the proximal ureter and renal anatomy after contrast administration.

Indications

- Evaluate poorly functioning renal tissue, urinary tract in the presence of calculi, obstruction, and poorly perfused renal tissue.

•••••••••••••
CLINICAL ALERT

◇ Obtain a signed, witnessed consent form.
◇ If ordered, renal function tests of serum and urine must be completed prior to retrograde pyelogram.
•••••••••••••

Expected Test Outcomes

Normal contour and size of kidneys, patent ureters.

Test Outcome Deviations

- Obstruction of urinary tract, tumors, calculi, congenital abnormalities, and reflux.

Interfering Factors

- Retained feces, barium and/or intestinal gas will obscure visualization of urinary tract.
- Metallic objects which overlie area of exam will interfere with organ visualization.
- Severe obesity adversely affects image quality.

Procedure

- Sedation and local anesthesia is required. A catheter is introduced into ureter via a cystoscope. Contrast media is injected and x-ray films are taken. Total exam time is generally less than 1 hour.

Nursing Role

Use nursing process model following pre-, intra-, and posttest care guidelines in Chapter 1. See page 8 for list of appropriate nursing diagnoses.

Nursing Diagnosis

- Knowledge deficit related to lack or possible misinterpretation of information provided about procedure or purpose.
- Anxiety and fear related to unfamiliarity with diagnostic procedure and equipment.
- Ineffective coping related to test outcome and inability to accept diagnosis of disease.
- High risk of injury related to iodine contrast use in procedure.

Pretest Care

- Assess for test contraindications: pregnancy, history of allergy to iodine.
- Explain exam purpose and procedure. No food is allowed for approximately 8 hours prior to study. Some labs also have fluid restrictions for patients undergoing retrograde pyelography. Make certain jewelry and metallic objects are removed from abdominal area. See Appendix A regarding contrast media precautions.
- A bowel prep may be necessary. This may consist of cleansing enemas and/or laxatives. Check protocol at laboratory performing the study.

Intratest Care

- Encourage patient to follow breathing and positional instructions.

Posttest Care

- Check vital signs for at least 24 hours.
- Provide plenty of fluids, food and rest after study.
- Record urine output and appearance for at least 24 hours. Hematuria and dysuria are common for several days after exam.
- Administer analgesics if necessary.
- Evaluate patient outcomes; provide support and counseling.

Rh Factors and Types

See Blood Groups and Types

Rheumatoid Factor   Blood
(RA Factor, RF)

This test measures the amount and quality of RF, a macroglobulin type of antibody found in rheumatoid arthritis.

Indications

- Diagnose rheumatoid arthritis (RA) and differentiate RA from other chronic inflammatory arthritis type disease.
- Monitor response to therapy.

Expected Test Outcomes

Results are reported as nonreactive or reactive/positive.
- Nonreactive: 0–39 IU/mL
- Weakly reactive: 40–79 IU/mL
- Reactive: > 80 IU/mL

Test Outcome Deviations

- Positive RF factor in rheumatoid arthritis.
- Elevated values occur in a variety of diseases other than rheumatoid arthritis, including lupus erythematosus, endocarditis, tuberculosis, syphilis, sarcoidosis, cancer, viral infections, diseases affecting the liver, lung, or kidney, Sjögren's disease, and in patients with skin and renal allografts.

Interfering Factors

- Results are higher in older persons and when multiple vaccinations and transfusions have been administered.
- Lipemic serum samples may prevent analysis if the rate nephelometry procedure is used.

Procedure

- Serum (5 mL) obtained by venipuncture according to specimen collection guidelines in Chapter 2.

Nursing Role

Use nursing process model following pre-, intra-, and posttest care guidelines in Chapter 1. See page 8 for list of appropriate nursing diagnoses.

Nursing Diagnosis

- Knowledge deficit related to lack of information provided about procedure and purpose and need for repeat testing.
- High risk of injury or infection related to venipuncture.

Pretest Care

- Assess the patient's knowledge base and note recent vaccinations and/or transfusion. If laboratory testing is by rate nephelometry, inform the patient that a fasting sample may be required. Check with laboratory.

Posttest Care

- Evaluate patient outcomes and counsel accordingly.

- Advise the patient that repeat testing is often necessary to evaluate response to long-term salicylate or other NSAID (non-steroidal anti-inflammatory drug) administration.

Routine Urinalysis (UA)

See Urinalysis

Rubella Antibody Tests   Blood

This test measures IgG and IgM antibody formation in regard to rubella virus, the causative agent of German measles, a usually mild disease unless it occurs in pregnant women.

Indications
- Determine immune status of patient.
- Confirm rubella infection.
- Identify potential carriers of rubella who may infect women of childbearing age such as health care workers.

Expected Test Outcomes
- Negative: Not immune to rubella virus.
- Positive: Immune to rubella virus.

Test Outcome Deviations
- A fourfold rise in titer between acute and convalescent samples indicates recent infection. Once a person has been infected, titer remains high for many years. This indicates immunity; repeat infections are rare. Immunization with rubella vaccine will cause production of rubella antibodies.
- Negative titers indicate no previous infection and lack of immunity.

Procedure
- Serum (5 mL) obtained by venipuncture according to specimen collection guidelines in Chapter 2. Follow-up testing may be required.

Nursing Role
Use nursing process model following pre-, intra-, and posttest care guidelines in Chapter 2. See page 8 for list of appropriate nursing diagnoses.

Nursing Diagnosis

- Knowledge deficit related to lack or misinterpretation of information provided about purpose, procedure and meaning of test outcomes.
- High risk of infection or injury related to venipuncture.

Pretest Care

- Assess patient's knowledge of test. Explain reason for testing and blood test procedure. Advise pregnant women that rubella infection in first trimester of pregnancy is associated with miscarriage, stillbirth, and congenital abnormalities.

Posttest Care

- Advise women of childbearing age if test is negative to obtain immunization before becoming pregnant.
- Vaccination during pregnancy is contraindicated.
- Advise patient with positive test that they are immune to further infection.

Schilling Test   Timed Urine Nuclear Procedure

This timed urine test evaluates ability to absorb vitamin B_{12} from the gastrointestinal tract, and is based on the anticipated urinary excretion of administered dose of radioactive vitamin B_{12}.

Indications

- Determine cause of vitamin B_{12} deficiency.
- Diagnose pernicious anemia and malabsorption syndromes.

Expected Test Outcomes

- Excretion of 7% or more of test dose of cobalt-tagged vitamin B_{12} in urine.

Test Outcome Deviations

- An abnormal low value (e.g., < 7%) or borderline (7%–10%) allows two interpretations; absence of intrinsic factor, or defective absorption in the ileum.
- When the absorption of radioactive vitamin B_{12} is low, the test must be repeated with intrinsic factor to rule out intestinal malabsorption (confirmatory Schilling test). If the urinary excretion then rises to normal levels, it indicates a lack of

intrinsic factor, suggesting the diagnosis of pernicious anemia. If the urinary excretion does not rise, malabsorption is considered the cause of the patient's anemia.

Interfering Factors

- The single most common source of error in performing the test is *incomplete collection of urine*. Some laboratories may require a 48-hour collection to allow for a small margin of error.
- Urinary excretion of B_{12} is depressed in elderly patients, diabetics, patients with hypothyroidism, and those with enteritis.
- Renal insufficiency and benign prostatic hypertrophy may cause reduced excretions of radioactive vitamin B_{12} and a 48- to 72-hour urine collection is advised.
- Fecal contamination of the urine may invalidate the test.

Procedure

- Patient must fast for 12 hours before test. (Breakfast is delayed 3 hours after vitamin B_{12} doses are administered.)
- A tasteless capsule of radioactive B_{12} labeled with ^{57}Co is administered orally by a nuclear medical technologist.
- Then a nonradioactive B_{12} is given by intramuscular injection by a registered nurse or nuclear medical technologist; usually 1000 µg of B_{12} is administered.
- Total urine is collected for 24–48 hours from time the patient receives the injection of vitamin B_{12}. Follow the procedure for timed 24-hour urine collection outlined in Chapter 2. Routine urine collection and disposal procedures are followed unless patient is also receiving therapeutic radiopharmaceutical treatment.

Nursing Role

Use nursing process model following pre-, intra-, and posttest care guidelines in Chapter 1. See page 8 for list of appropriate nursing diagnoses.

Nursing Diagnosis

- Knowledge deficit related to lack of or misinterpretation of information provided about purpose and procedure, and need for patient cooperation.
- High risk for injury/radiation hazard related to administration of radiopharmaceuticals.
- Potential for noncompliance related to patient/test requirements.

Pretest Care

- Explain purpose, procedure, fasting and collection of a 24-hour urine specimen. Water is permitted during fasting period. Record accurate weight.
- A random sample urine specimen is usually obtained before vitamin B_{12} doses are administered.
- Be certain patient receives the nonradioactive vitamin B_{12}. If the intramuscular dose of vitamin B_{12} is not given, radioactive vitamin B_{12} will be found in the liver, instead of the urine.
- Schedule bone marrow aspiration before the Schilling test, because the vitamin B_{12} administered in the test will destroy the diagnostic characteristics of the bone marrow.

Intratest Care

- Insure the patient remains fasting for 3 hours after the oral vitamin B_{12} has been given.
- Food and drink are permitted after the doses of vitamin B_{12} are given. Patient is encouraged to drink as much as can be tolerated during the entire test.
- Be certain that none of the urine is discarded.
- No laxatives or enemas are to be used during the test.

Posttest Care

- Evaluate patient outcomes and counsel appropriately.

Scrotal Ultrasound (Scrotal Sonogram), Testicular Sonogram, (Testicular Ultrasound)

Ultrasound Imaging

This noninvasive procedure images the testes and their surrounding structures.

Indications

- Identify and characterize testicular mass.
- Evaluate cause of testicular pain or potential changes resulting from testicular trauma.
- Evaluation of structural causes of male infertility and identify location of undescended testes.

Expected Test Outcome

Normal scrotal and testicular tissues.

Test Outcome Deviations

• Presence of space occupying lesions: tumors, abscesses, hematomas, hydrocele, gland enlargement or echo changes suggestive of inflammatory process, spermatocele, varicocele, infarct, undescended testes, and torsion as evidenced by lack of Doppler signal.

Procedure

• Penis is retracted and scrotum is supported on a rolled towel. After a coupling gel is applied to exposed scrotum, a hand-held transducer is gently moved across skin.
• Exam time is about 30 minutes.

Nursing Role

Use nursing process model following pre-, intra-, and posttest care guidelines in Chapter 1. See page 8 for list of appropriate nursing diagnoses.

Nursing Diagnosis

• Knowledge deficit related to lack of information or possible misinterpretation of information provided about procedure or its purpose.
• Anxiety and fear related to perception of diagnostic procedure as frightening or embarrassing.
• Ineffective coping related to test outcome and inability to accept diagnosis of testicular abnormality.
• Decisional conflict related to test outcome and potential for surgery.

Pretest Care

• Explain exam purpose and procedure. Assure patient that no radiation is employed and that test is painless.
• No preparation is required.

Posttest Care

• Remove or instruct patient to remove any residual gel from skin.
• Evaluate patient outcomes; provide support and counseling.

Sedimentation Rate (SED Rate)— Erythrocyte Sedimentation Rate (ESR)

Blood

This test measures the sedimentation rate or settling of RBCs and is used as a nonspecific measure of many diseases, especially inflammatory conditions.

Indications

- Monitor progress of inflammatory disease, rheumatic fever, rheumatoid arthritis, respiratory infections, and acute myocardial infarction.
- Diagnose occult disease.

Expected Outcomes

- Westergreen Method:
  Men: 0–15 mm/h
  Women: 0–20 mm/h
  Children: 0–10 mm/h

Test Outcome Deviations

- *Increases in* all collagen and autoimmune disorders, infections, myocardial infarcts, cancers, severe anemia, and heavy metal poisoning.
- *Decreased in* polycythemias, sickle cell anemia, spherocytosis, congestive heart failure, hypofibrinogenemia, and pyruvate kinase deficiency.

Interfering Factors

- Increased in pregnancy (after 12 weeks), postpartum, menstruation, drugs (heparin and oral contraceptives), age (very high in women 70–89); presence of cholesterol, globulins, and fibrinogen.
- Decreased with certain drugs (steroids, aspirin), presence of elevated WBCs, albumin and lipids; and decreased fibrinogen level in newborns; and blood allowed to stand before testing.

Procedure

- Anticoagulant venous sample of 7 mL is collected according to specimen guidelines in Chapter 2.
- Note any drugs patient is taking on lab slip or computer screen.

Nursing Role

Use nursing process model following pre-, intra-, and posttest care guidelines in Chapter 1. See page 8 for list of appropriate nursing diagnoses.

Nursing Diagnosis

- Knowledge deficit related to lack or misinterpretation of information provided about purpose and procedure.
- High risk for injury, bleeding, or infection following venipuncture.

Pretest Care

- Explain purpose and procedure.

Posttest Care

- Evaluate patient outcomes and counsel appropriately.
- Explain need for repeat testing to monitor progress and evaluate prescribed therapy.

Segmented Neutrophils

See Complete Blood Count (CBC)

Sickle Cell Test—   Blood
Hemoglobin S, Sickled ex

The test examines the RBCs for the sickle-shaped forms characteristic of sickle cell anemia and trait; detects the presence of hemoglobin S, an inherited recessive gene.

Indications

- Screen for sickle cells.
- Confirm sickle cell trait and diagnose sickle cell anemia.

Expected Test Outcomes

- Adult: No sickle cells present; no abnormal hemoglobin S present.

Test Outcome Deviations

- Positive test means hemoglobin S is present.
- Sickle cell trait: hemoglobin A/S; sickle cell anemia: hemoglobin S/S.

Interfering Factors

- False positives due to polycythemia, abnormal globulins, and other abnormal hemoglobins (Barts, Hgb C).
- False negatives in severe anemia or infants younger than 6 months.

Procedure

- A 5–7 mL venous blood sample (EDTA anticoagulent) added is obtained using specimen collection guidelines in Chapter 2.
- Note any blood transfusions 3–4 months prior on lab slip or computer screen.
- Electrophoresis is more specific and should be done in all positive Sickle ex scans.

Nursing Role

Use nursing process model following pre-, intra-, and posttest care guidelines in Chapter 1. See page 8 for list of appropriate nursing diagnoses.

Nursing Diagnosis

- Knowledge deficit related to lack or misinterpretation of information provided about purpose and procedure.
- High risk for injury, bleeding, or infection following venipuncture.
- Ineffective coping (individual or family) related to positive test outcomes.

Pretest Care

- Explain purpose and procedure of test.

Posttest Care

- Evaluate patient outcome and counsel and monitor appropriately. If outcomes reveal sickle cell anemia, plan care to treat fatigue, weakness, and severe joint and abdominal pain; prevention of infection and avoidance of high altitudes and cold climates.
- Advise genetic counseling if outcomes reveal sickle cell trait or anemia.

Signal Averaged Electrocardiogram (SAE)

See Electrocardiogram

Skin Tests   Special Study

*Allergy, Tuberculosis, Blastomycosis, Coccidiomycosis,
Histoplasmosis, and Toxoplasmosis*

Skin tests aid in diagnosis of both infectious and noninfectious disease when antigens are injected intradermally and interpreted based upon skin reactions.

Indications
- Screen high risk groups.
- Confirm sensitivity to allergens.
- Evaluate immune function.
- Determine susceptibility or resistance to specific infections.

Expected Test Outcomes
Negative or nonsignificant for sensitivity to allergens, tuberculosis, blastomycosis, coccidiomycosis, histoplasmosis, and toxoplasmosis.

Test Outcome Deviations
- *Positive o*r significant reactions for *allergens:* exaggerated response to allergy extracts such as house dust and pollen.
- *Positive* or significant reaction for *tuberculosis:* zone of induration 10 mm or more in diameter.
- *Positive* or significant reaction for *blastomycosis:* zone of erythema and induration by 5 mm or more in diameter.
- *Positive* or significant reaction to *coccidiomycosis:* zone of erythema and induration of 5 mm or more in diameter.
- *Positive* or significant reaction to *histoplasmosis:* zone of erythema induration of 5 mm or more in diameter.
- *Positive* or significant reaction to *toxoplasmosis:* zone of erythema area over 10 mm in diameter.

Procedure
- Most diagnostic skin tests are supplied in sterile kits. Follow manufacturer's instructions exactly. See Intratest Care.

Allergic disorders: Intradermal injection of specific allergens followed by reading of results. See manufacturer's directions.
Tuberculosis: Intradermal injection of tuberculin followed by reading of results in 48 hours.
Blastomycosis: Intradermal injection of blastomycin followed by

reading of results in 48 hours.

Coccidiomycosis: Intradermal injection of coccidioidin followed by reading of results in 24–72 hours.

Histoplasmosis: Intradermal injection of histoplasmin followed by reading of results in 24–48 hours.

Toxoplasmosis: Intradermal injection of toxoplasmin followed by reading of results in 24–48 hours.

∙∙∙∙∙∙∙∙∙∙∙∙∙∙
CLINICAL ALERT

◊ Falsely nonsignificant or negative test results do occur in all tests.

◊ Generally, a positive reaction is redness or swelling of more than 1 mm in diameter. A central area of necrosis is even more significant.

∙∙∙∙∙∙∙∙∙∙∙∙∙∙

Nursing Role

Use nursing process model following pre-, intra-, and posttest care guidelines in Chapter 1. See page 8 for list of appropriate nursing diagnoses.

Nursing Diagnosis

• Knowledge deficit related to lack or misinterpretation of information provided about purpose and procedure.
• High risk for injury or infection related to skin test procedure.

Pretest Care

• Explain purpose and procedure of skin testing.

Intratest Care

• For intradermal injection, cleanse skin (or inner aspect of forearm) and allow to dry. Stretch skin taut. Inject substance under skin so that a discrete pale elevation of skin—a wheel, 6–10 mm in diameter—is formed.
• Document site of test for follow-up reading of results.

Posttest Care

• Evaluate patient outcomes and counsel regarding outcomes.
• Read test results per specific skin test kit protocols. Examine in a good light. Inspect for redness and induration (hardening or thickening). Run your finger lightly over area of normal skin to indurated zone. Measure and record results.

Small Intestine X-Ray

See Gastric X-Ray

Sodium Blood and Timed Urine

See Electrolyte Studies

Spirometry

See Pulmonary Function Tests

Specific Gravity

See Urinalysis

Sputum Culture

Sputum

Sputum specimens are examined to identify organisms causing a respiratory illness.

Indications
- Diagnose disease of the lower respiratory tract.
- Determine antibiotic/drug sensitivity and course of treatment.
- Evaluate effectiveness of therapy or medication.

Expected Test Outcomes
- Negative culture for pathogenic organisms.

Test Outcome Deviations
- Pathogens indicative of tuberculosis, fungal infections, and causing pneumonia, bronchitis, and bronchiectasis.

Interfering Factors
- Antibiotics may cause false-negative cultures or may delay growth of organisms.
- Unsatisfactory sputum samples: contaminated specimens or "dry" specimens.

Procedure

- Sputum specimens must come from the bronchi. Postnasal secretions or saliva are unacceptable. Expectoration, ultrasonic nebulization, chest physiotherapy, nasotracheal or tracheal suctioning, or bronchoscopy are methods used to obtain sputum and bronchial specimens. See Intratest Care.

Nursing Role

Use nursing process model following pre-, intra-, and posttest care guidelines in Chapter 1. See page 8 for list of appropriate nursing diagnoses.

Nursing Diagnosis

- Knowledge deficit related to lack of or misinterpretation of information provided about purpose, procedure, and patient cooperation.
- Potential for noncompliance related to patient inability to adhere to collection guidelines.

Pretest Care

- Explain purpose, procedure, and all aspects of specimen collection. An early morning specimen produces the most organism-concentrated sample of deep pulmonary material. Instruct the patient regarding all aspects of collection.

Intratest Care

Expectorated Specimen Procedure
- Patient should clear nose and throat and rinse mouth prior to expectorating, then take several deep breaths, perform a series of short coughs, and then cough deeply and forcefully.
- Sputum should be expectorated into a sterile container with the proper preservative if it is called for. A 1–3-mL sample is adequate. Place sealed container into a leak-proof bag and transfer it to laboratory.
- Sputum specimens are usually not refrigerated. They should be taken to the laboratory immediately. Document pertinent information such as type of specimen, appearance, preservative, tests ordered, date and time of collection, and disposition of specimen.
- Document specimen appearance and patient's response to procedure. Label the specimen correctly.

Posttest Care

• Evaluate patient outcome and counsel appropriately.

• • • • • • • • • • • •
CLINICAL ALERT

◊ Use of ultrasonic nebulizers for sputum induction is recommended when cough is not productive. If this is the case, proper decontamination of nebulizer must be carried out.
◊ Do not suction without first consulting physician regarding this method of specimen collection.
• • • • • • • • • • • •

Standard Oral Glucose Tolerance Test (OGTT)

See Blood Glucose Tests

Stomach X-Ray

See Gastric X-Ray

Stool Analysis   Stool
Routine Fecal Studies

Fat, Meat Fibers, Occult Blood (Fecal Blood),
Parasites, Stool Culture

Analysis determines the various properties of stool such as color, as well as abnormal elements such as gross and occult blood, mucus, pus, parasites, and pathogenic organisms, tissue fragments, food residue, and fat.

• • • • • • • • • • • •
CLINICAL ALERT

◊ Assess appearance of feces before administration of barium, enemas, or laxatives.
• • • • • • • • • • • •

Indications

• Screen for colon cancer, asymptomatic ulcerative lesions of gastrointestinal (GI) tract, and unsuspected infections.
• Evaluate GI disorders in persons with diarrhea and constipation.
• Rule out in a routine stool culture presence of *Salmonella, Shigella, Compylobacter, Yersinia, Escherichia Coli* in the new-

born, and pure cultures of *Staphylococcus*.
- Use fat analysis as gold standard to diagnose malabsorption syndrome.

Expected Test Outcomes

MACROSCOPIC EXAMINATION	EXPECTED OUTCOMES
Amount	100–200 g/day
Color	Brown
Odor	Varies with pH of stool and depends upon bacterial fermentation and putrefaction.
Consistency	Plastic; not unusual to see seeds in a vegetable diet; small and dry in a high meat diet.
Size, shape	None
Gross blood, mucus, pus, and parasites	None

MICROSCOPIC EXAMINATION	EXPECTED OUTCOMES
Fat	Colorless, neutral fat (18%) and fatty acid crystals and soaps
Undigested food, meat fibers, starch, trypsin	None to small amount
Eggs and segments of parasites, yeasts, and leukocytes	None
Culture	Negative

CHEMICAL EXAMINATION	EXPECTED OUTCOMES
Occult blood	Negative

Test Outcome Deviations: Color

- The color of feces changes in disease states: *Yellow to yellow-green*—severe diarrhea; *black*—bleeding > 100 mL blood into upper GI tract; *pale or clay*—common bile duct blockage and pancreatic insufficiency; *red to pink*—bleeding from lower GI tract (blood streaks on outer surface), hemorrhoids, and anal problems; *bright red*—origin in stomach or duodenum, if transit time is very rapid.

Interfering Factors

- Stool darkens on standing.
- Color is influenced by diet (green with spinach; black with cherries and high meat; light with high milk and low meat; red with beets).
- Color is influenced by drugs: yellow-green (sterilization of bowel by antibiotics); black (iron, bismuth, charcoal); green (indomethacin), light white (barium, antacids); brown (anthrquinone); red (tetracylines in syrup); among many others.

···············
CLINICAL ALERT

◊ A complete dietary and medication history will help to differentiate abnormalities from interfering factors.
···············

Test Outcome Deviations: Mucus

- Mucus is abnormal and appears in conditions of parasympathetic excitation. Translucent mucus on surface of formed stool (in spastic constipation and emotionally disturbed patients). Bloody mucus clinging to stool (neoplasm, inflammation of rectum). Copious amounts of mucus of 3–4 L in 24 hours (villous adenomas) and mucus with pus and blood (ulcerative colitis, and ulcerating cancer). DucoLax suppositories cause excess mucus.

Test Outcome Deviations: Consistency

- Diarrhea mixed with mucus and red blood cells (cancer, amebiasis, cholera, typhus, and typhoid); diarrhea mixed with mucus and white cells (ulcerative colitis, shigellosis, salmonellosis, enteritis, and intestinal TB).
- Altered size and shape indicate motility or abnormalities in colon wall as a narrow ribbon-like stool (spastic bowel, partial obstruction); small, round, hard stools (habitual constipation); and severe fecal retention (huge impacted masses with a small amount of pasty stool is overflow).

Test Outcome Deviations: Cultures

- Presence of parasites, enteric disease-causing organisms, and viruses.

Test Outcome Deviations: Occult Blood

Positive test caused by cancer of colon and stomach; occurs in ulcerative colitis, diverticulitis, ulcers, and diaphragmatic hernia.

Interfering Factors for Blood in Stool

- Many foods and drugs may give false positive outcomes. Drugs include salicylates, steroids, indomethacin iron, massive doses, coumadin, vitamin C, boric acid, bromides, colchicine, alcohol, and iodine among others. Foods with hemoglobin and myoglobin enzymes and peroxidase activity such as meat and some vegetables.
- Other factors include bleeding hemorrhoids, menstrual contaminants, and vigorous exercise.

Test Outcome Deviations: Fecal Fat, Fatty Acids, Meat Fibers

- *Increases in fecal fat and fatty acids* with lack of lipase, enteritis and pancreatic disease, surgical removal and resection of part of intestine, and occurs in malabsorption syndromes (Crohn's disease and sprue).
- *Increased meat fibers* in malabsorption syndrome, pancreatitic dysfunction, and gastrocolic fistula (correlates with amount of fat excreted).

Interfering Factors

- Increased neutral fat may occur with use of rectal suppositories and oily perineal creams, castor and mineral oil; low-caloric dietetic mayonnaise and high fiber diet.

Procedures

- Collect feces in a dry, clean, urine-free container. Follow collection guidelines in Chapter 2. Laboratory will furnish instructions regarding preserving of specimen.
- Often parasite testing and stool culture will be ordered together. In this case, specimen is divided in half and one portion refrigerated for culture and one portion kept at room temperature for ova and parasites. A diarrhea stool will give good results. Stool passed into toilet bowl must *not* be used for cultures.

Procedure for Occult Blood

- Obtain a random stool specimen. Follow testing method (or instruct patient to do so) in manufacturer's directions exactly or results are not reliable. Use an aliquot from center of formed stool. A liquid stool may cause false negatives with filter paper methods. Time the reaction exactly.

∙∙∙∙∙∙∙∙∙∙∙∙∙∙
CLINICAL ALERT
for Blood in Stool Tests

◊ To be completely valid, the test employed must be repeated 3–6 times on different samples. Even one positive out of six should be considered positive and further evaluation is indicated.
∙∙∙∙∙∙∙∙∙∙∙∙∙∙

Procedure for Fat and Meat Fibers

• Collect a 24- or 72-hour specimen following specimen collection guidelines in Chapter 2. If a 72-hour specimen is ordered, each individual stool specimen is collected properly, identified and labeled, and sent immediately to the laboratory.

• If testing for meat fibers is ordered, specimens obtained with a warm saline enema or Fleet phosphosoda are acceptable.

∙∙∙∙∙∙∙∙∙∙∙∙∙∙
CLINICAL ALERT

◊ Specimens for fat testing obtained with mineral oil, bismuth, or magnesium compounds cannot be used.
∙∙∙∙∙∙∙∙∙∙∙∙∙∙

Nursing Role

Use nursing process model following pre-, intra-, and posttest care guidelines in Chapter 1. See page 8 for list of appropriate nursing diagnoses.

Nursing Diagnosis

• Knowledge deficit related to lack or possible misinterpretation of information provided about stool examination.

• Potential for noncompliance related to inability to follow directions for specimen collection and/or follow-up testing.

Pretest Care

• Explain purpose and diet requirements, procedure, interfering factors, and need to follow appropriate stool collection procedure. Diet prior to occult blood test is high residue (especially vegetables, fruit, bran cereals, and moderate amounts of peanuts and popcorn daily). Avoid foods with high peroxidase activity (red or rare meat, turnips, cauliflower, broccoli, cantaloupe, horseradish, and parsnips). Also, no alcohol, aspirin, or vitamin C 2 days before and during test period. For a 72-hour stool collection for fat, diet containing 60–100 g of fat, 100 g of protein, and 0.18 gm of carbohydrate is ordered for 6 days before and during the 72-hour test. If a test for meat fibers is ordered, a diet with an adequate amount of red meat is eaten for 24–72 hours before testing.

- List patient drugs that can affect test outcome on laboratory slip or computer screen.

Intratest Care

- Provide privacy during stool collection.
- Nursing observations and judgments regarding color, size, consistency, and presence of blood, mucus, parasites, and tissue and meat fibers are made.

Posttest Care

- Evaluate patient compliance and outcomes and counsel appropriately. Explain need for repeat or further testing if ordered.

· · · · · · · · · · · · · ·
CLINICAL ALERT

◊ At least three specimens, collected every other day or within a 10-day time frame, are needed to make a positive stool culture diagnosis.

◊ Inform patient that when a positive stool culture is diagnosed, personal contacts of the person and the convalescent patient should also have three negative stool cultures to prevent infection spread.

◊ See Appendix C for standards of critical (panic) values.
· · · · · · · · · · · · · ·

Stool Culture

See Stool Analysis

Stress Exercise Testing   Special Study
(Graded Exercise Tolerance Test)

Stress exercise testing measures heart efficiency during a controlled and monitored exercise session on a treadmill or ergometer.

Indications

- Diagnose ischemic heart disease and investigate angina, dysrhythmias, inordinate B/P elevation, valve competence, and pacemaker function.
- Measure functional capacity for work, sports, rehabilitation, or response to medical/surgical treatment, and set limits for an exercise program.
- Screen for asymptomatic coronary artery disease.

Expected Test Outcomes

- No significant symptoms, arrhythmias, or other EKG changes upon reading 85% of maximum heart rate predicted for age and sex. Exercise normally increases systolic BP but diastolic levels remain near normal.

Test Outcome Deviations

- Failure of systolic BP to rise, falling systolic BP, bradycardia, excessive tachycardia, ventricular tachycardia, multifocal PVCs, atrial tachycardia, second or third degree heart block, pacemaker failure, ST segment elevation or depression.
- Ventricular or supraventricular ectopics (not necessarily ischemic).
- Cyanosis, pallor, mottling, cold sweat, piloerection, ataxia, gallop rhythms, valvular regurgitation, abnormal cardiac impulse.

NOTE: Two findings strongly suggest an abnormality:

- Flat/downsloping ST segment depression of 1 mm or more for at least 0.08 second after the junction of the QRS and ST segments (J point).
- A markedly depressed J point with an upsloping but depressed ST segment of 1.5 mm below the baseline 0.08 second after the J point.
- Initial ST segment depression on resting EKG further depressed by 1 mm during exercise. Hypotension from exercise, 3 mm or greater ST depression, downsloped ST segment. Ischemic ST segments appearing within first 3 minutes of exercise and lasting 8 minutes into recovery period may indicate multivessel or left coronary artery disease. ST segment elevation can indicate dyskinetic left ventricular wall motion or severe transneural ischemia.

Interfering Factors

- False positive results can be from left ventricular hypertrophy, digitalis, ST segment abnormality at rest, hypertension, valvular heart disease, left bundle branch block, anemia, hypoxia, vasoregulatory asthenia, and Lown-Ganong-Levine syndrome.

Procedure

- A physician must be present.
- Electrode sites are shaved, prepped, and electrodes are secured with adhesive tape or a belt, according to leads chosen. A baseline EKG tracing is run and checked and BP is taken.
- The patient walks a treadmill or pedals an ergometer (if walking is difficult), while EKG, heart rate, and BP are continuously monitored. Treadmill starts at 1.7 mph at 10% incline. Every 3 minutes the speed and/or incline are increased (up to maximal speed of 3.3 mph and incline of 21%) as long as tolerated. Test is terminated when patient reaches maximal level or target heart rate or starts to experience severe dyspnea, fatigue, dizziness, claudication, angina level which previously caused patient to rest, ataxia, multiple PVCs, ST segment depression of 5 mm or more, exertional hypotension, decreasing heart rate with increased work, or severe anxiety.
- Recovery stage assessments are usually recorded in testing area until stable.

Nursing Role

Use nursing process model following pre-, intra-, and posttest care guidelines in Chapter 1. See page 8 for list of appropriate nursing diagnoses.

Nursing Diagnosis

- Potential for altered tissue perfusion (cardiopulmonary) related to physiological demands of stress test.
- Fear related to potential life-threatening event occurrence during stress testing.
- Potential for acute angina pain related to physiological demands of stress test.

Pretest Care

- Explain test purpose/procedure. Demonstrate equipment and provide for feedback/reassurance.
- Obtain legal consent form because of risk involved in test.
- Abstain from stressful exercise or stress testing for prior 12 hours. No eating/drinking, smoking, or nitroglycerine inges-

tion within 2 hours of test (may have a light breakfast sometimes).
- Administration of scheduled medications is physician's decision.
- Shave chest areas as necessary. Apply monitoring devices.
- Instruct patient to report symptoms/sensations.
- Walking shoes or tennis shoes, shorts, loose trousers/slacks, bra, front-button blouse are suggested attire. NO SLIPPERS OR PANTYHOSE.

Intratest Care

- Be alert to signs of anxiety, pain, hypotension, fatigue, dysrhythmias, and other signs and symptoms that would indicate a need to abort test.

Posttest Care

- Patient should not be discharged from test area until stable. No excessive exercise for rest of the day.
- Check vital signs upon return to nursing unit. Monitor for other untoward signs and symptoms and notify physician of these if necessary.
- Patient should rest for at least 1 hour. Avoid hot shower/bath for several hours. Resume diet.

••••••••••••
CLINICAL ALERTS

◊ Arrhythmias or symptoms may occur later after the test.
◊ Patients with unstable angina, congestive heart failure, or severe myocardial dysfunction are at greater risk during stress testing.

••••••••••••

Sugar (Glucose)

See Blood Glucose and Urinalysis

Syphilis Detection Tests—   Blood
VDRL, RPR, FTA-ABS, MHA-TP

These tests are done to diagnose syphilis, a venereal disease caused by *Treponema pallidum*. VDRL and RPR are nontreponemal (nonspecific) tests which determine the presence of reagin. FTA-ABS and MHA-TP are treponemal (specific) tests that determine presence of antibodies to *Treponema pallidum*.

Indications

- Evaluate infection with *Treponema pallidum*.
- Screen for and confirm syphilis.

Expected Test Outcomes

Nonreactive: negative for syphilis antibodies.

Test Outcome Deviations

- Infection with *Treponema pallidum* is indicated when both the screening and confirmatory tests are reactive.

Interfering Factors

- False-positive reactions: biologic false-positive (BFP) reactions can occur in nontreponemal tests in patients who abuse drugs, or who have diseases such as lupus erythematosus, mononucleosis, malaria, leprosy, or viral pneumonia; or who have been recently immunized; or rarely during pregnancy.
- False-negative reactions: non-treponemal tests may be negative early in the disease or during inactive or late stages of disease.
- Excess chyle in the blood interferes with test reaction. Avoid drawing the blood sample immediately after a meal.

Procedure

- Serum (5 mL) is obtained by venipuncture according to specimen collection guidelines in Chapter 2.
- Fasting is usually not required.

Nursing Role

Use nursing process model following pre-, intra-, and posttest care guidelines in Chapter 1. See page 8 for list of appropriate nursing diagnoses.

Nursing Diagnosis

- Knowledge deficit related to lack of knowledge or misinterpretation of information provided about purpose, procedure, and test outcome.
- High risk of injury or infection related to venipuncture.

Pretest Care

- Assess patient's knowledge of test and clinical history. Explain purpose and blood test procedure.

Posttest Care

- Evaluate patient outcomes and counsel appropriately. When test results contradict physician's opinion or patient's history, a repeat specimen should be submitted.
- Diagnosis of syphilis must be based on serologic tests as well as clinical history, a physical examination, and an epidemiologic explanation for source of infection.
- If result is a biologic false positive, assess patient's understanding that he/she does not have syphilis.

··············
CLINICAL ALERT

◊ Sexual partners of patients with primary, secondary, or early latent syphilis should be evaluated for signs and symptoms of syphilis and should have a blood test for syphilis. Social contacts of infants with symptomatic neonatal syphilis should be examined in a similar manner.
◊ After treatment, patients with early syphilis should be tested at 3-month intervals for 1 year. The reaction level declines in most patients followed for a year until little or no reaction is detected.

··············

T_3 Uptake

See Thyroid Function Tests

T_4

See Thyroid Function Tests

T and B Cell Lymphocyte Markers

See Immune Function Tests

Testosterone—Total and Free   Blood

This test measures testosterone production in both males (secreted by testes and adrenals) and females (secreted by ovaries and adrenals).

Indications

- Assess cause of premature puberty in boys and masculinity in females.

- Evaluate hypogonadism, cryptorchism in men.
- Detect ovarian and adrenal tumors in women.

Expected Test Outcomes

Testosterone—Total

Male: 270–1070 ng/dL
Female: 6–86 ng/dL

Testosterone—Free

AGE (Y)	PG/ML	
	MALE	FEMALE
20–29	19–41	0.9–3.2
30–39	18–39	0.8–3.0
40–49	16–33	0.6–2.5
50–59	13–31	0.3–2.7
> 60	9–26	0.2–2.2.

Test Outcome Deviations

- *Decreased totals in men* with pituitary failure, Klinefelter's syndrome, hypogonadism, hypopituitarism, orchidectomy, testicular failure, hepatic cirrhosis.
- *Increased total in men* in hyperthyroidism, androgen resistance, adrenal tumors, and precocious puberty.
- *Increased free in women* in hirsutism, polycystic ovaries, and masculinization.
- *Decreased free* in hypogonadism.

Interfering Factors

- Levels affected by radiopharmaceutical administration up to 24 hours prior to testing.
- Levels high in morning, drop up to 50% in males by midafternoon and drop 30% in females.

Procedure

- In women, five serum samples (10 mL) obtained by venipuncture following specimen collection guidelines in Chapter 2.
- In men, three serum samples (10 mL) obtained by venipuncture.
- Indicate sex and age on laboratory slip or computer screen.

Nursing Role

Use nursing process model following pre-, intra-, and posttest care guidelines in Chapter 1. See page 8 for list of appropriate nursing diagnoses.

Nursing Diagnosis

• Knowledge deficit related to lack or misinterpretation of information provided about purpose and procedure.
• High risk for injury related to venipuncture.

Pretest Care

• Explain purpose and procedure.

Posttest Care

• Evaluate outcomes, monitor, and counsel appropriately.

Thoracoscopy   Endoscopic Imaging

Thoracoscopy is the examination of the thoracic cavity with an endoscope.

Indications

• Evaluate and examine tumor growth, effusions, emphysema, inflammatory processes, pneumothorax.

Expected Test Outcomes

Normal thoracic tissues, parietal and visceral pleura, plueral spaces, thoracic walls, mediastinum, and pericardium.

Test Outcome Deviations

• Abnormal patterns include carcinoma (metastatic or primary), empyema, effusions, pneumothorax, inflammatory processes, diseases such as tuberculosis, coccidiomycosis, histoplasmosis.

Procedure

• A thoracoscopy is a surgical procedure and normally performed under general anesthesia. Chest tubes are usually placed; lung expansion and tube placement are confirmed by x-ray postoperatively.

Nursing Role

Use nursing process model following pre-, intra-, and posttest care guidelines in Chapter 1. See page 8 for list of appropriate nursing diagnoses.

Nursing Diagnosis

- Knowledge deficit related to lack or misinterpretation of information about procedure, purpose, and preparation.
- Anxiety related to experience of actual procedure or unknown diagnosis.
- Altered comfort related to pain, difficulty breathing.
- High risk for injury or infection related to presence of chest tube, incision.
- Ineffective breathing pattern related to pain of thorascopy procedure.

Pretest Care

- Explain test purpose, procedure.

· · · · · · · · · · · · · ·
CLINICAL ALERT

◊ Obtain and check for properly signed and witnessed surgical permit and check proper pre-op lab work, x-rays, EKG, and other required tests.
· · · · · · · · · · · · · ·

- Patient should be fasting at least 8 hours preoperatively.
- Start IV line if ordered and administer preoperative medications.
- Document care accurately.

Posttest Care

- Administer postanesthesia care per institutional guidelines.
- Monitor vital signs, respiratory status, lung sounds, and arterial blood gases (if ordered); report abnormalities promptly. Check chest tube patency, drainage, bubbling, fluctuation of fluid level in drainage tubing, and record. Report abnormalities promptly.
- Administer pain medication as needed; monitor respiratory status closely. Assist patient to cough and deep breathe frequently. Encourage ambulation and leg exercises frequently.
- Document care accurately.

· · · · · · · · · · · · · ·
CLINICAL ALERT

◊ Watch for signs of increasing respiratory problems or bleeding and report promptly.
◊ **DO NOT CLAMP CHEST TUBES UNLESS SPECIFICALLY ORDERED.** Clamping them may produce a tension pneumothorax.
◊ Sudden sharp pain, together with dyspnea, uneven chest wall movement, tachycardia, anxiety, and cyanosis may signal development of a pneumothorax—notify physician immediately.

· · · · · · · · · · · · · ·

Thrombin Time (TT) and Thrombin Clotting Time (TCT)

See Coagulation Studies

Thyroid Function Tests   Blood

T$_4$ Total, T$_3$ Uptake (UP), Free Thyroxine Index (FTI) T$_7$, Thyroid Stimulating Hormone (TSH) Thyrotropin

These tests are indirect and direct measurements of thyroid status and are initially done to diagnose thyroid dysfunction and disease in persons with tremor, muscular weakness, congestive heart failure, and hyponatremia.

Indications

• Determine thyroid function and rule out hypo- and hyperthyroidism.
• Evaluate thyroid replacement therapy.

Expected Test Outcomes

• *T$_4$ total:* 4.5–11.5 µg/dL
• *T$_3$ uptake (UP):* 26–39% In spite of its name, this test has nothing to do with the actual T$_3$ blood level. T$_3$ UP and true T$_3$ are entirely different tests.
• *Free thyroxine index (FTI) T$_7$:* 1.2–4.5 µg/dL. American Thyroid Association now recommends the term thyroid-hormone bonding ratio rather than FTI.
• *TSH:* Adult 0.5–6.0 milli IU/L
  Children 0.4–7.0 µ IU/L

Test Outcome Deviations: T₄ Total

- *T₄ total increases* in hyperthyroidism, thyrotoxicosis, Hashimoto's disease, subacute thyroiditis (first stage), and liver disease.
- *T₄ total decreases* in cretinism, myxedema, hypothyroidism, subacute thyroiditis (third stage), hyponatremia caused by nephrosis, cirrhosis, and malnutrition.

Interfering Factors

- *T₄ total increases* in certain drugs (estrogen, birth control pills, TSH, thyroid extract, D-thyroxine, anticonvulsants, heroin and methadone, media and pregnancy, and iodine contrast.

Test Outcome Deviations: T₃ Uptake

- *T₃ uptake increases* in hyperthyroidism, nephrosis, severe liver disease, deficiency of thyroxine-binding globulin, desiccated thyroid and thyroxine therapy, and severe acidosis.
- *T₃ uptake decreases* in hypothyroidism, treatment for hypothyroidism, acute intermittent porphyria, excess thyroxine-binding globulin, estrogen producing tumors, and subacute thyroiditis.

Test Outcome Deviations: FTI

- *FTI increases* in hyperthyroidism.
- *FTI decreases* in hypothyroidism.
- *TSH increases* in adults with primary hypothyroidism, Hashimoto's thyroiditis, some non-thyroid sick patients, TSH antibodies.

Test Outcome Deviations: TSH

- *TSH decreases* in hyperthyroidism, thyrotoxicosis due to thyroiditis, secondary pituitary or hypothalmic hypothyroidism, nonthyroid sick patients, acute psychiatric illness, liver disease, malnutrition, Addison's, acromegaly.

Interfering Factors, TSH

- Decreases during treatment with T₃, aspirin, corticosteroids, heparin, and during first trimester pregnancy.
- Increases during treatment with lithium, potassium iodide TSH injection, and dopamine.

Procedures

T$_4$ Total Procedure

- Blood (5 mL) obtained by venipuncture following specimen collection guidelines in Chapter 2.
- To get a valid T$_4$ total, thyroid treatment should be discontinued one month before testing.

T$_3$ Uptake Procedure

- Blood (at least 2 mL) obtained by venipuncture according to specimen collection guidelines in Chapter 2.

FTI (T$_7$) Procedure

- This is a calculated value: $T_4 \times T_3UP\% / 100 = FTI$ (T$_7$).

Nursing Role

Use nursing process model following pre-, intra-, and posttest care guidelines in Chapter 1. See page 8 for list of appropriate nursing diagnoses.

Nursing Diagnosis

- Knowledge deficit related to lack or misinterpretation of information provided about purpose and procedure of thyroid tests.
- High risk of infection or injury related to venipuncture.

Pretest Care

- Explain purpose, procedure, and interfering factors of thyroid function tests.
- Obtain medical history, concentrating on thyroid prescriptions and over-the-counter drugs and drugs that affect testing. See Interfering Factors.

Posttest Care

- Evaluate patient outcomes, monitor and counsel appropriately. Explain that if outcomes are abnormal, further blood testing that is more specific for thyroid functions will be required.

Thyroid Scan   Nuclear Medicine Scan Imaging

This nuclear test measures the uptake of radioactive iodine (^{123}I) or technetium ^{99m}TC by the thyroid and is done to evaluate size, shape, and function of thyroid tissue.

Indications

- Establish thyroid origin of neck masses and evaluate functional activity of thyroid nodules.
- Monitor effectiveness of thyroid therapies (medication, radiation, or surgery) and check the thyroid response to drugs through suppression or stimulation tests.

Expected Test Outcomes

Normal or evenly distributed concentration of radioactive iodine; normal size, position, shape, site, weight, and function of thyroid; absence of nodules.

Test Outcome Deviations

- *Decreased uptake*: Cancer of the thyroid, hypothyroidism, and Hashimoto's disease.
- *Increased uptake*: Hyperthyroidism, Grave's disease, and autonomous nodules.

Interfering Factors

- Ingested iodine and contrast diagnostic substances interfere up to 6 months.

Procedure

- The patient swallows radioactive iodine in either a tasteless capsule or liquid form or has the radionuclide injected intravenously (for ^{99m}Tc).
- After administration, the neck area is scanned at 10 minutes when ^{99m}Tc is used and at 2–6 hours when ^{123}I is used.

Nursing Role

Use nursing process model following pre-, intra-, and posttest care guidelines in Chapter 1. See page 8 for list of appropriate nursing diagnoses.

Nursing Diagnosis

- Knowledge deficit related to lack of or misinterpretation of information provided about purpose, procedure and administration of radiopharmaceutical.
- High risk for injury/radioactive hazard related to radiopharmaceutical injection.
- High risk for infection at IV site following injection of radiopharmaceutical.

Pretest Care

- Explain purpose, procedure, and record accurate weight. Reassure regarding safety of nuclear scan. See Nuclear Medicine Scans: Overview.
- Advise that iodine intake is restricted for at least 1 week before test. Consult with physician regarding restricted substances: some thyroid drugs, multiple vitamins, some oral contraceptives, cough medicines, and iodine-containing foods.
- Test is contraindicated in pregnancy.
- Schedule this test before x-ray using iodine contrast and before thyroid or iodine containing drugs are given.
- Assess for iodine allergy and consult with physician regarding these data.

Intratest Care

- Provide support and reassurance.

Posttest Care

- Evaluate patient outcomes and counsel and monitor as necessary.
- Check IV site of radiopharmaceutical injection for infection.
- Body fluids and secretions can be routinely disposed of unless the patient is also receiving therapeutic doses of radioactive meds.
- Pregnant staff and visitors are to avoid prolonged contact for 24–48 hours after radioactive administration.
- Document any patient problems that may have occurred during the procedure.

Thyroid Sonogram— Thyroid Ultrasound, Thyroid Echogram

Ultrasound Imaging

This noninvasive procedure is used to visualize and measure the thyroid gland. Because this procedure does not require the use of radiation of any sort, it is the diagnostic method of choice in pregnant patients.

Indications

- Identification and characterization of masses (cysts or solids) and infectious processes.
- Gland measurement to monitor therapeutic outcomes.
- Guidance during biopsy or cyst aspiration.

Expected Test Outcomes

Normal anatomy of thyroid and surrounding structures.

Test Outcome Deviations

- Gland enlargement and presence of space occupying lesions: cysts, solid masses such as adenomas or nodules, hematomas, abscesses.

Interfering Factors

- Very small lesions may escape detection.
- Sonography cannot differentiate benign from malignant lesions.
- Parathyroid lesions or other extra-thyroid masses may not be differentiated from intra-thyroid lesions.

Procedure

- A coupling medium, generally a gel, is applied to exposed hyperextended neck in order to promote transmission of sound. An ultrasound transducer is slowly moved across the skin. Exam time is about 30 minutes.

Nursing Role

Use nursing process model following pre-, intra-, and posttest care guidelines in Chapter 1. See page 8 for list of appropriate nursing diagnoses.

Nursing Diagnosis

- Knowledge deficit related to lack or possible misinterpretation of information provided about purpose and procedure.
- Anxiety and fear related to unfamiliarity with diagnostic procedure and equipment.
- Ineffective coping related to test outcome and inability to accept diagnosis of thyroid disease.
- Decisional conflict related to test outcome and potential for interventional procedures.

Pretest Care

- Explain exam purpose and procedure. Assure patient that no radiation is employed and that test is painless. Explain that a coupling gel will be applied to skin. Although couplant does not stain, advise patient to avoid wearing non-washable clothing. Advise patient to remove any neck chains prior to procedure.

• No other preparation is necessary.

Posttest Care
• Remove or instruct patient to remove any residual gel from skin.
• Evaluate patient outcomes; provide support and counseling.

•••••••••••••
CLINICAL ALERT

◊ Patient must agree to and sign a surgical permit prior to performance of an ultrasound guided biopsy or other interventional procedure.

•••••••••••••

Thyroid Stimulating Hormone (TSH)

See Thyroid Function Test

Thyroxine (T$_4$)

See Thyroid Function Tests

TORCH Test   Blood

TORCH (acronym that stands for toxoplasma, rubella, cytomegalovirus, and herpes simplex) identifies agents frequently implicated in congenital infections of the newborn and confirmed by the demonstration of specific IgM-associated antibodies in the infant's blood.

Indications
• Evaluate possible congenital infection with one or more of the TORCH agents.

Expected Test Outcomes
Negative for antibodies to toxoplasma, rubella, cytomegalovirus, and herpes simplex.

Test Outcome Deviations
• Presence of IgG antibodies suggests transfer of antibodies from mother to newborn.
• Presence of IgM antibodies suggests congenital infection.

Interfering Factors

- TORCH screen is not always useful because antibody production may not occur in detectable amounts early in the infection.
- TORCH is more useful in excluding a possible infection than proving etiology.

Procedure

- A venous or cord blood sample of 3 mL is obtained following specimen collection guidelines in Chapter 2. Follow agency policy for collection of cord blood.

Nursing Role

Use nursing process model following pre-, intra-, and posttest care guidelines in Chapter 1. See page 8 for list of appropriate nursing diagnoses.

Nursing Diagnosis

- Knowledge deficit related to lack or misinterpretation of information provided about purpose and procedure.
- High risk of injury or infection following venipuncture or cord sampling.

Pretest Care

- Assess parent's knowledge of test.
- Explain blood collection procedure to parent.

Posttest Care

- Evaluate patient outcomes, monitor and counsel appropriately.

Total Iron-Binding Capacity (TIBC)

See Iron Tests

Toxoplasmosis (TPM)   Blood
Antibody Tests; Indirect Fluorescent
Antibody (IFA) Tests

This test is done to diagnose toxoplasmosis, a disease caused by the sporozoan parasite *Toxoplasma gondii*, by detecting antibodies to the parasite; test helps to differentiate toxoplasmosis from infectious mononucleosis.

Indications

- Evaluate toxoplasma infection in patients with enlarged lymph glands and other infectious mononucleosis-like symptoms.
- Assess pregnant women who may be asymptomatically infected.
- Evaluate immunocompromised patients in whom the disease may become very serious or fatal.

Expected Test Outcomes

Negative for antibodies to *Toxoplasma gondii*.

Test Outcome Deviations

- Any titer in a newborn is abnormal.
- Titer 1:16–1:64 indicates past exposure. Titer 1:256 indicates recent exposure or current infection. Titer 1:1024 significant; may reflect active disease, and rising titers are of greatest significance.

Interfering Factors

- False positives in patients with high rheumatoid factor levels.
- False negatives in immunocompromised patients because of their impaired ability to produce antibody.
- Newborns may have antibody received from their mothers and should be retested.

Procedure

- Serum sample (5 mL) is obtained by venipuncture following specimen collection guidelines in Chapter 2.

Nursing Role

Use nursing process model following pre-, intra-, and posttest care guidelines in Chapter 1. See page 8 for list of appropriate nursing diagnoses.

Nursing Diagnosis

- Knowledge deficit related to lack of or possible misinterpretation of information provided about procedure and purpose.
- High risk of injury or infection related to venipuncture.

Pretest Care

- Assess patient's knowledge of test, clinical symptoms, and possible exposure to the parasite through uncooked meat or cat feces. Explain purpose and blood test procedure.

- Advise patient that test for infectious mononucleosis may also be performed.
- Advise pregnant women that parasite can be passed to fetus, causing neurological and eye problems, and may lead to fetal death.

Posttest Care

- Advise patient if results are not significant that test may be repeated to check for rising titer.
- Diagnosis of congenital toxoplasmosis may require additional test procedures, such as demonstration of the parasite in cerebral spinal fluid and detection of nonmaternal antibodies in the serum.

Transferrin

See Iron Tests

Triglycerides

See Cholesterol Studies

Tuberculosis

See Skin Tests

Tumor Markers   Blood

Acid Phosphatase (Prostatic Acid Phosphatase—PAP), Lactate Dehydrogenase (LDH), Neuron Specific Enolase (NSE), Alkaline Phosphatase (ALP), Immunoglobulin-Monoclonal Proteins (M Protein), Human Chorionic Gonatropin, (HCG), Calcitonin (CT), CA 15-3, β-2-Microglobulin, HLA Antigen, Prostate Specific Antigen [PSA], CA 125, and CA 19-9 Tissue, Polypeptide Antigen (TPA), α-Fetoprotein (AFP), and Carcinoembryonic Antigen (CEA)

These tests measure the presence of substances produced and secreted by tumor cells that are found in the serum of patients with specific types of carcinomas.

Indications

- Detect malignancy to pinpoint the tissue of origin.
- Assess extent of tumor or disease and estimate progress.

- Evaluate tumor burden, change, and follow clinical course.
- Monitor effect of therapy on recurrence.

Expected Test Outcomes

Enzymes

- Prostatic acid phosphatase (PAP)
    Adult: 0–3.1 mg/mL
    Child: 8.6–12.6 U/mL
    Newborn: 10.4–16.4 U/mL
- Lactate dehydrogenase (LDH): increased isoenzymes I and II.
- Neuron-specific enolase (NSE): normal staining.
- Alkaline phosphatase (ALP)
    Adult: 30–85 U/mL
    Child: <2 y—85–235 U/mL
    2–21 y: 30–200 U/mL

Hormones

- Human chorionic gonatropin, (HCG)
    Male: <2.5 IU/L
    Female: nonpregnant <5.0 IU/L
    Postmenopausal: <9.0 IU/L
    Pregnancy: peaks in 10 weeks gestation
- Calcitonin (CT) (malignant C-cell tumor): <14–19 pg/mL

Proteins

- CA 15-3 antigen (metastic breast): <22 μ/mL.
- β 2-microglobulin (HLA antigen system) 4–12 mg/mL.
- Prostate specific antigen (PSA): 0–4 ng/mL.
- CA 125 (ovarian cancer) (glycoprotein): 0–35 U/mL
- CA 19-9 (pancreatic-hepatobiliary cancer): <37 U/mL
- Tissue polypeptide antigen (TPA): 80–100 U/L in serum—may also be detected in urine, washings, and effusions.
- Immunoglobulins, monoclonal protein: Absent.

Oncofetal Antigens

- α-Fetoprotein (AFP): 10 ng/mL.
- Carcinoembryonic antigen (CEA): 0–2.5 ng/mL; (10 ng in smokers).

Test Outcome Deviations: PAP

- *High significant levels* in metastic prostate cancer; level drop in 3–4 days after successful surgery treatment and 3–4 weeks after estrogen administration. *Moderate level elevation* in benign prostate hypertrophy. *Also elevated* in leukemia and cancer metastic to bone; *noncancer elevation* in osteoporosis, renal osteopathy, hepatic cirrhosis, pulmonary embolism, prostate surgery, massage and chronic prostatis, Paget's disease, Gaucher's disease, and hyperparathyroidism.

Interfering Factors, PAP

- Drugs that elevate androgens and clofibrate. Drugs that decrease fluorides, phosphatase, oxalates, and alcohol.
- False high levels after prostate, rectal exam, or instrumentation (ie, cystoscopy).

Test Outcome Deviations: LDH

- *Cancer*—acute lymphocytic leukemia, non-Hodgkin's lymphoma, Ewing's sarcoma, neurobastomic carcinoma of testes. *Noncancer*—cellular injury/hemolysis, myocardial infarction, hepatic diseases; see Cardiac Enzyme tests.

Interfering Factors, LDH

- Hemolysis of blood can cause false positives. Ascorbic acid decreases; several drugs increase, (aspirin, alcohol, narcotics, and anesthetics).

Test Outcome Deviations: NSE

- *NSE increases* in neuroblastomas, small cell lung carcinoma, medullary carcinoma of thyroid, pancreatic islet cell and Wilm's tumors, and phenochromcytoma.

Test Outcome Deviations: ALP

- *ALP increased levels: Cancers*—osteosarcoma, hepatocellular, metastic to liver, primary or secondary bone tumors. *Noncancer*—Paget's disease, nonmalignant liver disease, normal pregnancy, healing fractures, hyperparathyroidism.
- *Decreased levels*: hypoparathyroidism, malnutrition, scurvy, pernicious anemia.

Interfering Factors, ALP

- Drugs false elevations in albumin from placenta tissue, allopurinol, antibiotics, colchicine, fluoride, indomethacin, INH, oral contraceptives, probenecid. Drugs decrease in arsenicals, cyanide, oxalates, zinc salts, nitrofuradantion.

Test Outcome Deviations: HCG

- *HCG increases in cancer*: gestational trophoblastic tumors, seminomatous and nonseminomatous testes cancer, and less valuable in lung, GI, lymphoproliferative diseases. *Noncancer*: increased hydatidiform mole, neoplasm of stomach, colon, pancreas, lung and liver, multiple pregnancy. Levels double every 48 hours during early pregnancy.
- *HCG decreases* in 48 hours in ectopic pregnancy and abortion. Not increased in endodermal sinus tumors.

Test Outcome Deviations: CT

- *CT increases in cancer*: medullary carcinoma of thyroid, lung, breast, pancreas, hepatoma, and renal cell carcinoid. *Noncancer*: Zollinger-Ellison syndrome, pernicious anemia, chronic renal failure, pseudohypoparathyroidism, alcoholic cirrhosis, Paget's disease, and pregnancy.

Test Outcome Deviations: CA 15-3

- *CA 15-3 increases in cancer*: metastic breast greatly elevated. Limited in primary or small tumor burden of breast cancer as levels not as high. *Noncancer*: elevations in benign breast or ovarian disease.
- *Levels decrease* with therapy and *increase* rise after therapy suggests progressive disease.

Test Outcome Deviations: β-2 Microglobulin

- β-2 *microglobulin increases in cancer*: multiple myeloma, other B-cell neoplasms, lung cancer, hepatoma, breast cancer. *Noncancer*: *increased level* in ankylosing spondylitis and Reiter's syndrome.

Test Outcome Deviations: PSA

- *PSA increases in cancer*: prostate, the higher the level, the greater the tumor burden. Successful surgery, chemotherapy, or radiation causes marked reduction in levels. *Noncancer*: benign prostatic hypertrophy, prostate massage, and prostate surgery; prostatitis.

Test Outcome Deviations: CA 125

- *Ca 125 increases in cancer*: epithelial ovarian, fallopian tube, endometrium, endocervix, liver, pancreas.
- *Less increase:* colon, breast, lung. Progressive decline in positive therapy response—a rise after successful therapy may pre-

dict recurrent tumor. *Noncancer*: pregnancy, advanced stage of endometriosis, cirrhosis, severe liver necrosis, peritonitis, other GI and pancreas diseases.

Interfering Factors, CA 125

- False positive in pregnancy and normal menstruation.

Test Outcome Deviations: CA 19-9

- *CA 19-9 increases in cancer*: pancreas and hepatobiliary cancer primarily. Mild elevation in gastric and colorectal. *Noncancer*: pancreatitis, cholecystis, cirrhosis, gallstones, and cystic fibrosis (minimal elevations).

Test Outcome Deviations: TPA

- *TPA increases in cancer*: gastrointestinal, genitourinary tract, breast, lung, thyroid. *Noncancer*: hepatitis, cholangitis, cirrhosis, diabetes, pneumonia, or urinary infections.

Test Outcome Deviations: Monoclonal Protein

- *Monoclonal protein in cancer*: multiple myeloma, macroglobulinemia, amyloidosis, B cell lymphoma, multiple solid tumors. *Noncancer*: cold agglutin disease, mixed cryoglobulin, Sjögren's syndrome, Gaucher's disease, lichen myedematosus, cirrhosis, renal failure, sarcoid.

Interfering Factors, Monoclonal Protein

- Drugs that may give false increases: gammaglobulins, hydrolazines, INH, dilantin, tetanus toxoid and antitoxin, and procainamide. Indicate on lab slip if patient received vaccines or immunizations in past 6 months.

Test Outcome Deviations: AFP

- *AFP increases in cancer*: primary hepatocellular cancer, embryonal cell carcinoma of testes (never elevated in pure seminoma), yolk sac tumors, teratocarcinoma, gastric, renal, and lung; can cross react with LH, increases in gonadal failure. *Noncancer*: fetal distress and death, neural tube defects, hepatitis, primary biliary cirrhosis, partial hepatectomy, ataxia telangectasia, Wiskott-Aldrich syndrome, multiple pregnancy, and abortion.

Test Outcome Deviations: CEA

- *CEA increases in cancer*: primarily colon cancer, especially monitoring persistent metastic or recurrence of colon cancer. Other—lung, metastic breast, pancreas, prostate, ovary, bladder, limbs, neuroblastoma, leukemia, osteogenic carcinoma. *Noncancer*: inflammatory bowel disease, pancreatitis, bronchitis, pulmonary infections, colonic polyps, chronic renal failure, cirrhosis, peptic ulcers, fibrocystic breast disease. Most levels decline with remission of disease.

Procedure

- A venous blood sample (10 mL) is usually obtained for most tests. Refer to Chapter 2 for specimen collection guidelines.
- For PAP, note on lab slip if patient has had prostatic exam or instrumentation of prostate within 24 hours.
- Note other specific test preparations under interfering factors.
- Follow specific lab procedure for handling of each specimen.

Nursing Role

Use nursing process model following pre-, intra-, and posttest care guidelines in Chapter 1. See page 8 for list of appropriate nursing diagnoses.

Nursing Diagnosis

- Knowledge deficit related to lack or misinterpretation of information provided about purpose, procedure, and repeat testing.
- High risk of injury, infection, or bleeding related to venipuncture.
- Potential ineffective coping, individual or family, related to unexpected test outcome of diagnosis of cancer.
- Potential for denial related to not believing test results.

Pretest Care

- Assess patient's knowledge of test. Explain purpose and procedure of blood test and prepare patient for possible test outcome indicative of cancer.

Posttest Care

- Evaluate outcomes, monitor, and provide counseling regarding unexpected test outcome and possible "bad news."

Ultrasound Overview

Diagnostic ultrasound makes use of high frequency sound waves (inaudible) that are directed into soft tissue recesses in the body, producing an echo when the sound meets a tissue boundary. The echo information is returned to the ultrasound apparatus which uses computer technology to process the echo information. A visual pattern of "dots" is formed, representing the strength and position of the echoes. Different tissues will produce echoes of varying strengths, providing evidence of various pathologies. In most instances, representative images from the ultrasound study are recorded for documentation.

Ultrasonography is generally noninvasive, no radiation used, relatively quick to perform, only limited patient preparation required, and believed to be safe and without measurable bio-effects.

Applications for diagnostic ultrasound include gynecologic, obstetric, abdominal, and vascular; echocardiography, evaluate masses, infections, and other disturbances within the testes, breasts, thyroid/parathyroid, eye, fetus, and prostate.

Upper GI Study

See Gastric X-Ray

Uric Acid

See Kidney Function Tests

Urinalysis Routine (UA)   Urine

Color, Appearance, Specific Gravity, pH, Odor,
Microscopic Examination of Sediment (Bacteria, Casts,
Red Blood Cells, White Blood Cells, Crystals), Glucose, Ketones,
Blood, Protein, Bilirubin, Urobilinogen

Urinalysis is the means of determining the various properties of urine as well as any abnormal constituents, revealed by microscopic examination of the sediment and clinical determinations.

Indications

- Use as screening in routine physical examination, prehospital admission, and presurgical procedures.
- Diagnose kidney and urinary tract infections and metabolic diseases not related to urinary system.

Expected Test Outcomes

Adult Values

GENERAL CHARACTERISTICS AND MEASUREMENTS	CHEMICAL DETERMINATIONS	MICROSCOPIC EXAM OF SEDIMENT
Color: pale yellow to amber	Glucose: negative	Bacteria: negative; Casts negative: occasional hyaline casts
Appearance: clear to slightly hazy	Ketones: negative	Red blood cells: negative or rare
Specific gravity: 1.015–1.025 with a normal fluid intake	Protein: negative	Crystals: negative
Infant: < 2 y specific gravity: 1.001–1.018	Bilirubin: negative or 0.2 mg/dL	White blood cells: negative or rare
pH: 4.5–8.0— av. person has pH of 5–6	Urobilinogen: 0.1–1.0 units	Epithelial cells: few
Odor: aromatic	Nitrate: for bacteria: negative	

Test Outcome Deviations: Appearance

- Cloudy urine may indicate presence of pus, red blood cells, or bacteria due to urinary tract infection, or may be normal.

Interfering Factors, Appearance

- Foods, urates, phosphates, or vaginal contamination, and degree of hydration or dehydration may affect appearance.

Test Outcome Deviations, Color

- Abnormal-colored urine may be due to presence of red blood cells (smoky), bilirubin (brown or yellow-green); fever (orange); melanotic tumor or Addison's (black), alkaptonuria (black); and porphyria (port wine).

Interfering Factors, Color

- Color darkens on standing, certain foods (red/beets), medications (all colors), physiologic factors (stress/clear), excessive exercise (red), large fluid intake and alcohol (straw).

Test Outcome Deviations, Odor

- Abnormal odor may be due to foods (asparagus, garlic) medications (estrogen), bacteria (putrid), ketones (sweet), and in PKU (musty, mousey), tyrosenemia (cabbage, fishy), maple sugar urine disease (burnt sugar), and oathouse urine disease (brewery odor).

Test Outcome Deviations, Specific Gravity

- *Low specific gravity* 1.000–1.010 may occur in CF, diabetes insipidus due to no ADH, glomerulonephritis, and pyelonephrets, and medications(diuretics), and increased fluid intake.
- *High specific gravity* above 1.025 may be due to elevated protein levels, low fluid intake, excessive water loss, fever, vomiting, diarrhea, and medications such as stool softeners, increased secretion of ADH, and diabetes mellitus.
- *Fixed specific gravity* of 1.010 that does not vary from specimen to specimen indicates severe renal damage.

Interfering Factors, Specific Gravity

- Radiopaque contrast used in urologic x-ray, manitol and dextrose infusion, detergent residue, and cold specimen temperature may affect.

Test Outcome Deviations: pH

- *Acid urine* (pH less than 7) is found in acidosis, uncontrolled diabetes, diarrhea, dehydration, starvation, respiratory disease with retention of carbon dioxide, medication (mandelamine and ammonium chloride), foods (cranberry and pineapple juice and vitamin C).
- *Alkaline urine* (pH above 7) bacteriuria, urinary tract infections, chronic renal failure, respiratory disease with loss of carbon dioxide, pyloric obstruction, renal tubular acidosis, and medications (salicylate intoxication and some antibiotics).

Test Outcome Deviations: Microscopic Examination of Sediment

- *Bacteria* in urinary tract infections, *red cell casts* in acute infections, glomerulonephritis, *broad casts* in serious kidney, *white cell casts* in pyelonephritis. *Epithelial casts* in tubular renal epithelial cell disease, tubular damage. *Granular casts* in renal parenchymal disease. *Hyaline casts* in acid urine, high salt content, *squamous epithelial cells* in tubular disease. *Leukocytes* (WBCs) in most renal disorders, urinary tract infections, and pyuria.

Interfering Factors, Microscopic Examination

- Traumatic catheterization, alkaline urine, vaginal discharge, and improper specimen collection.

Test Outcome Deviations:
Bacteria/Nitrate or Leukocyte Esterase Dipstick Methods

- Positive results indicate pyuria and reliable indication of bacteriuria.

∙∙∙∙∙∙∙∙∙∙∙∙∙∙
CLINICAL ALERT

◊ The presence of bacteria indicates the need for urine culture. Notify physician and record results in the patient's record.
∙∙∙∙∙∙∙∙∙∙∙∙∙∙

Interfering Factors, Bacteria/Nitrate

- Vaginal discharge, trichomonas, parasites, and heavy mucus can cause false positives.
- Azo-dye metabolites, high specific gravity, and ascorbic acid may affect test outcomes.

Test Outcome Deviations: Glucose/Sugar

- *Increased amounts,* (glycosuria) in diabetes mellitus, brain injury, myocardial infarction, infections lowered renal threshold: (positive *urine* glucose, normal *blood* glucose)

Interfering Factors, Glucose

- Pregnancy, lactation, stress, excitement, ketonuria, testing after a heavy meal, IV glucose, some meds (ascorbic acid, keflex); use of deteriorated reagent strips and inappropriate procedures.

Test Outcome Deviations, Ketones

- *Increased* amounts, *ketonuria*, occur in acute illness, anorexia, starvation, fasting, diarrhea, prolonged vomiting, and following anesthesia.

Interfering Factors, Ketones

- Dietary increased fat and protein, low carbohydrate, and many drugs (insulin, pyridium, isopropyl alcohol, bromosulfophelein (BSP) phenosulfophalein (PSP) compounds, levadopa and many others) may affect test outcomes.

·············
CLINICAL ALERT

◊ The presence of ketones is a crisis situation. In diabetics: suggests inadequate glucose control; in nondiabetics: indicates a small amount of carbohydrate metabolism and excessive fat metabolism.
·············

Test Outcome Deviations: Blood

- *Presence of blood,* (hemoglobinuria) occurs in excessive burns and crushing injuries, transfusion reaction, febrile intoxication, chemical agents, snake venom, malaria and other parasites, hemolytic disorders (sickle cell anemia), hypertension, paroxysmal hemoglobinuria, kidney infarction, disseminated intravascular coagulation (DIC), and favabean sensitivity.
- *Increased red blood cells,* (hematuria) occurs in lower urinary tract infections, benign prostatic hypertrophy, glomerulonephritis, SLE, hemophilia, benign familial hematuria, and urologic cancer.

Interfering Factors, Blood

- Strenuous exercise, smoking, menstruation contamination, and many drugs (ascorbic acid, antibiotics toxic to kidney, anticoagulants, salicylates, bromides, copper, iodine) may affect test outcomes.

·············
CLINICAL ALERT FOR BLOOD

◊ The appearance of blood in urine is one of the early indications of renal disease.
◊ Any instance of hematuria should be rechecked on a freshly collected specimen. If hematuria is still present, further evaluation must occur. Notify physician.
·············

Test Outcome Deviations, Proteins

- See Protein in alphabetical list for this item.

Test Outcome Deviations, Bilirubin

- Bilirubin is always abnormal and warrants further investigation.
- Urine bilirubin is negative in hemolytic disease.
- *Increased levels* occur in hepatitis and liver disease (due to

infections or toxic agent), obstructive biliary tract, and parenchymal injury.

Interfering Factors, Bilirubin

- Light exposure to specimen and many drugs affect test outcomes.

Test Outcome Deviations: Urobilinogen

- See Liver Function Tests in alphabetical list for this item.

Procedure

- Collect fresh random midstream urine specimen following collection guidelines in Chapter 2.
- Take reagent strip (a chemically impregnated paper strip) from container; be sure container is kept tightly closed when not in use and never remove preservative desiccant.
- Dip reagent strip in well-mixed urine and remove immediately. If left too long in urine, the chemical will dissolve.
- Blot off excess urine on strip to avoid chemical becoming mixed on multiple test strips.
- Compare each reagent area with the corresponding color chart on the bottle using the specified time period (seconds) on the bottle. Precise timing is essential for accurate results.
- Read manufacturer's directions carefully each time procedure is done, as manufacturers frequently revise directives.

Nursing Role

Use nursing process model following pre-, intra-, and posttest care guidelines in Chapter 1. See page 8 for list of appropriate nursing diagnoses.

Nursing Diagnosis

- Knowledge deficit related to lack of or possible misinterpretation of information provided about procedure, purpose, and preparation.
- Potential for noncompliance related to inability to follow directions for specimen collection.

Pretest Care

- Explain purpose and procedure and need to follow appropriate urine collection procedures.
- List patient drugs that can affect test outcome on laboratory slip or computer screen.

Intratest Care

• Provide privacy during urine collection.
• Testing procedure usually done by the nurse or other trained person.

Posttest Care

• Evaluate patient compliance in specimen collection, outcomes, and counsel appropriately. If urine is red color, do not assume drug causation. Check urine for hemoglobin.
• Explain need for follow-up testing if indicated.
• Record test results and, if abnormal results, inform physician.

....
CLINICAL ALERT

◊ See Appendix C for standards of critical (panic) values.
....

Urine Culture
Urine

Urine culture is done to identify the specific causative organisms in suspected infections of kidneys, ureter, bladder, and urethra.

Indications

• Isolate microorganisms that cause clinical infections of urinary tract.
• Evaluate effectiveness of medication therapy for existing urinary infection.

Expected Test Outcomes

• Adults: Negative less than 10,000 organisms/mL of urine. Any bacteria found are either contaminates from the skin or invading pathogens.
• Pediatric: Same as adult. Urine cultures of *E. coli* are not definitely significant unless they contain more than 100,000 organisms/mL urine.

Test Outcome Deviations

• Bacterial count of 100,000 or more per mL urine indicates infection.
• A significant titer of the following organisms in urine is considered pathogenic: *E. coli, Enteroccus, Gonococcus, Klebsiella*

species, *Mycobacterium tuberculosus, Proteus* species, *Pseudomonas aeruginosa, Staphylococcus supraphyticus, Trichomonas vaginalis*, and *Candida albicans* and other yeasts.

Interfering Factors
- Urine may be diluted with a reduction in bacteria colony count when patients have been forcing fluids.
- Specimens not taken to laboratory immediately or refrigerated (no longer than 2 hours). Urine at room temperature allows growth of many organisms.
- Not following collection procedure accurately.
- Urine contaminated during collection may lead to false test results. Sources of contamination include: hair from perineum, bacteria from beneath prepuce in men, bacteria from vaginal secretion, vulva, or urethra in women, and bacteria from hands, skin, or clothing.

Procedure
- Collect a clean catch midstream specimen according to specimen collection guidelines in Chapter 2.
- Two successive clean catch specimens should be collected in order to be 95% certain that true bacteria is present and results are not a result of urine contamination.
- Specimens collected should preferably be an early morning one when bacterial count is likely to be highest (urine concentrated) and before initiating antibiotic therapy.
- A sterile urine specimen may be collected by urethral catheterization, suprapubic catheter aspiration, or directly from an indwelling catheter (see Chapter 2 guidelines for collection of that type of specimen).

Nursing Role
Use nursing process model following pre-, intra-, and posttest care guidelines in Chapter 1. See page 8 for list of appropriate nursing diagnoses.

Nursing Diagnosis
- Knowledge deficit related to lack of or possible misinterpretation of information about procedure and purpose.
- Potential noncompliance related to not understanding or following clean catch midstream urine collection procedure.
- Knowledge deficit related to the significance of positive test

outcomes and the need for patient education in relation to adherence to followup medical therapy.

Pretest Care

- Assess patient's knowledge of the test, and medication usage. Explain purpose and procedure for collection of clean catch midstream urine specimen.
- Hold antibiotics or sulfonamide until after specimen has been collected if possible. Monitor patient's temperature to correlate with potential urinary tract infection.
- Provide patient with necessary supplies, including sterile specimen container and antiseptic sponges.

Intratest Care

- Usually, patient collects this specimen if able to do so physically and comprehends directions. If not, nurse collects specimen. Provide privacy during collection procedure.
- Use good handwashing before and after collection of specimen (also gloves if nurse collects the urine).
- Label specimen as follows: patient's name, suspected clinical diagnosis, method of collection, precise time collected, whether fluids forced or on IV therapy, and any specific antibiotics or sulfonamides administered.
- Send the specimen to the laboratory immediately.

··············
CLINICAL ALERT

◇ If collection for cytomegalovirus, the urine should be kept at room temperature until taken to the viral laboratory, as refrigeration destroys the urine.
··············

Posttest Care

- Counsel patient in relation to any life-style changes necessary to prevent further urinary tract infections, such as proper perineal cleansing after bowel and urinary elimination, avoiding tight, restricting clothes (pants, hose), and drinking sufficient fluids.

··············
CLINICAL ALERT

◇ See Appendix C for standards of critical (panic) values.
··············

Urobilinogen

See Liver Function Tests

Urodynamic Studies   Special Study

Cystometrogram (CMG), Urethral Pressure,
Recal Electromyogram (EMG), Cystourethrogram

These tests identify abnormal voiding patterns in persons with
incontinence and inability to void normally.

Indications
- Evaluate incontinence, abnormal voiding patterns, dysuria,
  enuresis, infections.
- Measure status of neuroanatomic connections between spinal
  cord, brain, and bladder.
- Evaluate neurogenic bladder dysfunction and assess neu-
  ropathies such as multiple sclerosis, diabetes, tabes dorsalis.

Expected Test Outcomes
- Normal bladder sensations of fullness, heat, cold. Normal
  adult bladder capacity: 400–500 mL; residual urine less than
  30 mL; desire to void: 175–250 mL; sensation of fullness:
  350–450 mL; strong uninterrupted stream.
- Normal voiding pressure and muscle coordination.
- Normal rectal EMG readings; urethra pressure profile readings normal.

Interfering Factors
- Inability of patient to cooperate (as in disorientation).

Test Outcome Deviations
- Motor/sensory deficits of pelvic floor muscle and/or internal sphincter and disturbed muscle coordination.
- Detrusor muscle hyperreflexia (due to upper or lower motor
  neuron lesions such as cerebrovascular aneurysm, Parkinson's, multiple sclerosis, cervical spondylosis, spinal cord
  injury above conus medullaris).
- Hyperreflexia—caused by benign prostatic hypertrophy or
  stress urge incontinence.
- Detrusor areflexia—difficulty voiding without a residual vol-

ume because of inadequate detrusor muscle response to innervation. (Causes: trauma, spinal arachnoiditis, birth defects, diabetes, phenothiazines, reduced estrogen levels in menopause.)

Procedure

- Instruct patient about purpose of the test, collection, and refrigeration of specimen. Follow specimen collection guidelines in Chapter 2. See Appendix E for standards for timed urine collection.

Cystometrogram Procedure

Residual urine is measured with an indwelling catheter after patient voids. Flow rate, pressures, and urine amount is recorded during voiding. After cystometric exam, cholinergics or anticholinergics may be injected to check bladder response to these drugs. When this is done, the first cystometric is used as a control and a second cystrometric is done about 30 minutes after drug injection.

Rectal EMG Procedure

Electrodes are placed next to the anus and grounded on the thigh, or a needle electrode may be placed into the periurethral striated muscle. Measurements of EMG activity during voiding produce a recording of urine flow rate.

Urethral Pressure Profile Procedure

A specially designed catheter coupled to a transducer records urethral pressures as it is slowly withdrawn.

Cystourethrogram Procedure

This study evaluates stress incontinence in females, bladder wall and urethral abnormalities, tumors, reflux, and posttraumatic urine extroversion. X-ray contrast material is instilled via catheter until the bladder fills. X-rays of the patient in several positions are taken. Catheter is then removed and more x-rays of contrast medium being voided through urethra are taken (voiding cystourethrogram).

Nursing Role

Use nursing process model following pre-, intra-, and posttest care guidelines in Chapter 1. See page 8 for list of appropriate nursing diagnoses.

Nursing Diagnosis

- Knowledge deficit related to lack of or misinterpretation of information provided about purpose, procedure, and need for patient cooperation.
- High risk for injury or infection related to urodynamic procedures.

Pretest Care

- Explain testing purpose, procedure, and collection of specimens. Be sensitive to cultural, social, sexual, and modesty issues.
- Describe expected sensations of urgency, discomfort, pressure.
- Instruct patient not to move or change position unless requested to do so.

••••••••••••••
CLINICAL ALERT

◊ Obtain a properly signed and witnessed consent form if needed.
••••••••••••••

Intratest Care

- Provide emotional support and privacy.
- Observe patient during the procedure for sensations/perceptions.
- Assist as necessary with the actual procedure, collection, and refrigeration of specimens.

Posttest Care

- Encourage increased oral fluid intake.
- Explain that minor burning/discomfort is normal immediately after the test.
- Instruct patient to notify physician STAT if fever, chills, tachycardia, faintness occur—watch for hypotension, also.

••••••••••••••
CLINICAL ALERTS

◊ Patients are not sedated because they must verify sensations and perceptions.
◊ Preexisting urinary tract infections can precipitate a septic reaction.
◊ Some patients with cervical spine cord lesions may experience autonomic reflexia that produces hypertension, severe

headache, bradycardia, flushing, and diaphoresis. Propantheline bromide (Pro-Banthrine) can alleviate these symptoms.

••••••••••••••

Vanillylmandelic Acid (VMA)—(Catecholamines, 3-Methoxyl-4-Hydroxymandelic Acid)

Timed
Urine

This test measures the excretion of urinary catecholamines, the substances formed by the adrenal medulla.

Indications

- Evaluate hypertensive person suspected of having pheochromocytoma.
- Diagnose malignant neuroblastoma in children.

Expected Test Outcomes

- Vanillylmandelic acid: 2–11 µg/mL/24 h or up to 35.4 µmol/24 h.
- Catecholamines:
  Epinephrine: 0–15 µg/24 h or 0.0–81.9 nmol/24 h.
  Norepinephrine: 0–100 µ/24 h or 0–591 nmol/24 h.
  Metanephrine: 0.25–0.8 mg/24 h or 1.27–4.06 µmol/24 h.
  Dopamine: 65–400 µg/24 h or 424–2612 nmol/24 h.

Test Outcome Deviations

- *Increased VMA* found in pheochromocytoma, neuroblastomas, strenuous exercise, severe stress, depressive neurosis, manic-depressive disorders.
- *Increased catecholamines* found in pheochromocytoma, neuroblastomas, progressive muscular dystrophy, myasthenia gravis, Guillain-Barré syndrome, acute intermittent porphyria, and carcinoid syndrome.

Interfering Factors

- Increased levels of VMA are caused by starvation (test should not be scheduled while patient NPO) and many foods such as tea, coffee, cocoa, chocolate, vanilla, fruit—(especially bananas, fruit juice) food containing artificial flavoring or coloring, food containing licorice.
- Many drugs cause false positive, such as antihypertensives, antibiotics, vasopressors, epinephrine (Adrenalin), amino-

phylline, insulin, levodopa, isoproponol, chlorpromazine (Thorazine), vitamins B and C.
• Decreased levels of VMA are caused by alkaline urine, uremia, radiographic iodine contrast agents, specific drugs.

Procedure

• Collect urine for 24 hours in a clean container. See timed specimen collection guidelines in Chapter 2, and Appendix E for standards. Keep specimen refrigerated, preservative in container. The pH of the urine collection should be below 3.0, if not, more hydrochloric acid may be required.
• Note drugs patient is taking on lab slip or computer screen.

Nursing Role

Use nursing process model following pre-, intra-, and posttest care guidelines in Chapter 1. See page 8 for list of appropriate nursing diagnoses.

Nursing Diagnosis

• Knowledge deficit related to lack of information or possible misinterpretation of information provided about procedure, purpose, and preparation.
• Potential for noncompliance related to inability to adhere to collection guidelines.
• Impaired adjustment related to denial, disbelief, and nonacceptance of health changes and significance of test outcome.

Pretest Care

• Restrict diet from foods listed in Interfering Factors for 3 days (2 days prior to testing and day of the test).
• All drugs should be discontinued for 3–7 days before testing with physician's permission.
• Assess patient compliance.
• Assess patient knowledge base prior to explaining test purpose and procedure.

Intratest Care

• Rest and adequate food and fluids are encouraged.
• Avoid strenuous exercise and stress as both can cause increases in VMA levels.
• Accurate test results depend on proper collection, preservation, and labeling. Be sure to include test start and comple-

tion times. Record drugs the patient must take on the lab slip or computer screen.

Posttest Care

• Evaluate patient outcome. Provide counseling and support as appropriate.

Very Low Density Lipoproteins (VLDL) and Low Density Lipoproteins

See Cholesterol Tests

White Blood Cell Count (WBCs)

See Complete Blood Count (CBC)

Wound Culture and Sensitivity (C&S)

Wound Exudate

Would cultures are obtained to isolate pathogenic microorganisms (both aerobic and anaerobic) in patients with suspected wound infections.

Indications

• Identify specific microorganisms in a wound infection, especially when amount, consistency, or odor of drainage changes significantly.
• Determine appropriate antibiotic therapy for an infection or evaluate effectiveness of treatment.
• Document absence of transmissible microorganisms, especially when isolation procedures are considered.

Expected Test Outcomes

Negative for pathogenic microorganisms, only normal flora found on microscopic examination.

Test Outcome Deviations

• Wound infected with pathogenic microorganisms such as: *Pseudomonas, Staphylococcus aureus*, Proteus, Bacteroides, Klebsiella, *Fusobacterium, Serratia, Streptococcus* D, *Nocardia,*

Actinomyces, Mycobacterium species, *Escherichia coli, Clostridium perfringens,* and *Candida.*

Interfering Factors

- Antibiotic medications (either systemically or topically) administered prior to taking of culture.
- Cleansing of wound or irrigation with an antiseptic solution prior to culture may kill the organism and produce a false negative culture report.

Procedure

- Use universal precautions.
- Wound culture may be obtained by aspiration, tissue biopsy, and swab culture. Nurses usually only do the swab culture, so this procedure will be emphasized.
- Use a culture kit containing a sterile cotton swab or a polyester-tipped swab and a tube with a culture medium.
- Wear sterile gloves, if excess amount of purulent drainage.
- Preparation of wound prior to culture:
  Cleanse to risk introduction of extraneous microorganisms into specimen—if you culture only the *external exudate,* you may miss the real cause of the infection. If *moderate-to-heavy* drainage, irrigate with normal saline until all visible debris has been washed away—use a sterile gauze to absorb excess normal saline and expose culture site.

  In *chronic wounds* such as decubitus ulcers, debridement may be necessary—remove loose necrotic tissue and culture clean area of granulation tissue. *If a wound has been treated with a topical antibiotic or antiseptic,* clean thoroughly to remove the residual prior to culture.

  Incision wounds may require removing of a few staples or sutures to gain access to wound infection (or use needed biopsy procedures).

Nursing Diagnosis

- Knowledge deficit related to lack of information or possible misinterpretation of information provided about procedure, purpose, and preparation.
- High risk of infection related to microorganisms in wound exudate.
- Potential for impaired social interaction if culture report identifies an organism requiring patient isolation and possible decreased social interaction.

Pretest Care

- Explain test purpose and procedure for obtaining the culture specimen.
- Hold antibiotics or sulfonamides until after specimen has been collected. If these drugs have been given, identify them on the lab slip.

Intratest Care

- Use universal precautions and sterile aseptic techniques.
- Remove swab from sterile collection container. Separate margins of deep wounds with thumb and forefinger, swab into pus of infected wound. Press and rotate swab several times over clean wound surface to extract tissue fluid containing potential pathogens. Avoid touching swab to intact skin at wound edges to prevent introducing superficial skin organisms into culture. Take culture in such a way that exposure to oxygen is minimized with aerobic specimen collection. Preferably, use two swabs and transfer each one to its own sterile medium tubes.
- After obtaining culture, insert swab into sterile container—break swab and discard top portion (area contaminated with gloved hand). Seal container and avoid touching inner surface of container.

Nursing Role

Use nursing process model following pre-, intra-, and posttest care guidelines in Chapter 1. See page 8 for list of appropriate nursing diagnoses.

- Label specimen with patient's name, date and time collected, anatomical site or specific source of specimen (chest incision wound), type of specimen (abscess fluid, granulatous tissue), exam requested, patient's diagnosis, any topical or systemic medication currently administered, and isolation status.
- Transport specimen to the laboratory immediately after testing (within 30 minutes) or check with laboratory regarding refrigeration or proper storage. (Anaerobic organisms often are not refrigerated.)

Posttest Care

- Reapply sterile dressing to wound if required prior to wound culture.
- Notify physician of any positive results so appropriate antibiotic therapy can be initiated. A preliminary report is

usually available in 24 hours; however, it usually requires 48–72 hours for growth and identification of organism.

....
CLINICAL ALERTS

◊ After appropriate antibiotic therapy, repeat cultures may be done to assess for resolution of infection.
◊ Counsel patient regarding test outcome deviations and the need to use good techniques, including hand washing, when performing self-care to the wound.
....

X-Ray Overview

X-rays are invisible electromagnetic images capable of penetrating through all but very dense substances. After a beam of x-rays is directed at a specific body part, a pattern of varying x-ray intensities will result. This pattern is imaged on a television screen (as in fluoroscopy), on film, or a variety of digital high-test display devices such as CT. Computerized tomography (CT or CAT) is a computer-enhanced method of displaying cross-sectional images of the body. CT involves radiation and often requires administration of contrast agents (iodine or barium used most often). (See Appendix A for standards and precautions when using contrast.)

....
CLINICAL ALERT

◊ Whenever the body is exposed to radiation, there is risk that tissues will be damaged. Radiation damage is manifested in cells of exposed individual (hair loss, reddened skin, increased risk of cancer), and is termed *somatic effects*. When reproductive organs are exposed to radiation, damage may be manifested in the offspring of the exposed individual. These effects are termed *genetic*.
◊ Radiation exposures are cumulative (meaning they add up); thus, every precaution must be taken to limit radiation doses. The greatest potential hazards for radiation injury are the tissues of the embryo and developing fetus. Good medical management will prevent unnecessary radiation exposure due to repeated x-ray studies.
◊ Women who are pregnant or could be pregnant should avoid x-ray studies which expose pelvic or abdominal regions.

When x-rays are performed on other body parts (for example, teeth), a protective lead apron should be placed over woman's abdomen/pelvis during x-ray exposure.

◊ When it is necessary for nurses to assist with high-risk, medically unstable, uncooperative persons or comatose patients during the procedure, lead aprons and other protective gear should be worn by all staff.

• • • • • • • • • • • • •

Appendix A
• • • • • • • • • • • • • •

Standards for
Contrast Media Precautions

Nursing Practice Standard

The nurse follows agency protocols, appropriate nursing standards for diagnostic procedures involving contrast media, and uses nursing process model for pretest care, procedural patient/family education, intratest care, and posttest monitoring and evaluation.

Radiopaque contrast substances such as iodine and barium are used to temporarily change the amount of x-ray energy that body structures (hollow organs of GI tract or blood vessels) will absorb (enhancement process).

• • • • • • • • • • • • • •
CLINICAL ALERT

◇ Iodized oil and barium are used for GI tract structures, but **only** water soluble iodine agents can be used for injection into the blood stream.
◇ All contrast agents have the potential for causing reactions mild to severe.

• • • • • • • • • • • • • •

Frances Talaska Fischbach: QUICK REFERENCE TO COMMON LABORATORY AND DIAGNOSTIC TESTS. © 1995 J.B. Lippincott Company

Nursing Process With Procedures Using Iodine Contrast Media

Pretest Care

- Assess for certain conditions that contraindicate the use of iodine such as syphilis, pheochromocytoma, multiple myeloma, pregnancy, asthma, chronic obstructive pulmonary disease, renal failure, and long-term steroid use.
- Assess for known iodine sensitivity (allergy). Some of the newer non-iodine contrast agents may be used safely. Inform radiology department of the above medical condition or allergies prior to test.
- Schedule x-ray procedures that require injection of contrast agents into the blood stream prior to barium studies.
- Prior to contrast administration, patient should be NPO for several hours (see agency protocol) to prevent nausea, vomiting, severe reactions, and aspiration of gastric contents.

Intratest Care

- Monitor patient closely for side effects/allergy reactions during and following contrast administration. Reactions happen quickly and usually within minutes of administration of media; reactions occur in anyone, but most likely in those between 20–49 years of age.

Posttest Care

- Assess for reactions, monitor vital signs.
- Flush contrast media from body by drinking fluids posttest, unless contraindicated.
- Inform patient/family regarding unexpected test outcomes and counsel appropriately.

Nursing Process With Procedures Using Barium Contrast Media

Pretest Care

- Assess for contraindications such as suspected bowel perforation and ulcerative colitis.
- Schedule barium tests after x-ray or ultrasound studies of abdominal or pelvic area.
- If patient has an ostomy, notify radiology department as patient preparation and testing procedures may vary depending upon location and extent of ostomy.

- Consult with radiology department for pretest preparation: upper intestines require NPO 8–12 hours prior; large intestine usually requires bowel cleansing with laxative.

Intratest Care

- Assist patients as necessary during test procedure, especially elderly, confused, pediatric, and those requiring close medical monitoring.
- Barium sulfate is administered orally or as an enema to visualize structures of alimentary canal. Most posttest complications relate to eliminating barium from GI tract.

Posttest Care

- Follow agency posttest care protocols—constipation can be prevented by giving adequate fluids and mild laxatives as necessary.
- Avoid narcotics posttest as these slow elimination.
- Assess for impactions, especially the elderly, which may first present as symptom of fainting.
- Observe stool color posttest. Normally, stool will be very light, but should return to normal color within 2 days. Persistently light stools should be reported to physician.
- Inform patient/family regarding unexpected test outcomes and counsel appropriately.

Appendix B
....

Standards for Intravenous Sedation Precautions

Nursing Practice Standard

The nurse follows agency protocols and appropriate nursing standards when caring for patients receiving IV sedation for diagnostic tests and procedures.

During more complex diagnostic procedures, patients frequently receive IV sedation. The nurse may administer as well

as monitor patient's response to these drugs even though anes-
thesiologist or attending physician assumes responsibility.

- Prior to procedure, establish IV line and keep open with the ordered IV solution.
- Monitor vital signs, EKG and pulse oximetry in pre-, intra- and posttesting according to established guidelines. Results should be documented.
- Assess pain and discomfort levels at frequent intervals. Arrhythmias should be promptly reported and treated if necessary. Frequent respiratory assessments are mandatory. If oxygen saturation drops below acceptable levels (90%), sedation may need to be held or reversed (Naloxone and Mazicon are two reversal agents) and oxygen therapy may be necessary until SaO_2 levels, vital signs and cardiac rhythms are acceptable.
- Prepare for emergency situations by having resuscitation equipment and supplies readily available.
- Administer sedation/medication per physician's discretion, frequently, often in incremental doses. The two most commonly used drugs are diazepam (Valium) and midazolom (Versed).
- Record any unexpected outcomes and follow-up interventions.

Appendix C
. . . .

Standards for Unexpected Test Outcome: Critical Values

NURSING PRACTICE STANDARD

The nurse notifies and collaborates with the physician immediately when the patient's verified test results occur outside the limits of expected outcome (critical values), as any sudden change in the patient's laboratory test values could become an imminent life-threatening situation.

Test	Low Unexpected Outcome	High Unexpected Outcome
Blood-Hematology and Coagulation Studies		
Hematocrit	<15 vol %	>60 vol %
Hematocrit (neonate)	<33 vol %	>70 vol %
Hemoglobin	<5 g/dL	>18 g/dL
Hemoglobin (neonate)	<9.5 g/dL	>22 g/dL
WBC	<1500/Cu mm	>15,000/Cu mm
Platelet count	<30,000/Cu mm	>1,000,000/Cu mm
Platelet count (ped.)	<20,000/Cu mm	>1,000,000/Cu mm
Prothrombin time	None	40 sec or 3× control level
Activated partial thromboplastin time	None	>90 sec
Bleeding time	—	>15 min
Chemistry—Electrolytes		
Bilirubin	—	>12 mg/dL
Bilirubin (neonate)	None	>10 mg/dL
Calcium	<6 mg/dL	>14 mg/dL
Creatinine kinase	None	>3–5x normal
Glucose	<40 mg/dL	>700 mg/dL
Glucose (neonate)	<30 mg/dL	>300 mg/dL
Magnesium	<0.5 mEq/L	>4.5 mEq/L
Osmolality	<240 mOsm/kg	>321 mOsm/kg
Phosphorous	<1 mg/d	None
Potassium	<2.5 mEq/L	6.5 mEq/L
Potassium (neonate)	<2.5 mEq/L	>8.0 mEq/L
Sodium	<120 mEq/L	>160 mEq/L
Blood–Gases Arterial		
CO (carbon monoxide)	—	>10%
HCO_3	<10 mmol/L	>40 mmol/L
O_2 content	<10%	—
O_2 saturated	<75%	—
pCO_2	<20 mm Hg	> 60 mm Hg
pH	<7.2	>7.6
pO_2	<40 mm Hg	—

Test	Low Unexpected Outcome	High Unexpected Outcome
Venous		
HCO_3	<10 mmol/L	>40 mmol/L
O_2 saturated	<40%	>85%
pCO_2	<20 mm Hg	>60 mm Hg
pH	<7.2	>7.6
Microbiology—Serology and Other		
Blood culture/smear		Positive
CSF culture/gram stain		Positive
Bacterial antigens		Antigen detected
Blood cross match		Incompatible
Blood parasites—malaria		Present
Stool culture		Positive for Salmonella, Shigella, or Campylobacter
Specific Organisms—Blood		
Tuberculosis		Positive acid-fast stain or culture
Hepatitis		Positive
Syphilis		Positive
AIDs		Positive
CSF—total protein	Low–none	High > 45 mg/dL
CSF—glucose	Low <80% of blood level	
CSF—WBC	Low–none	High–increased
CSF—blasts or malignant cells	Low–none	High–increased
Urine—Glucose		Strongly positive >1000 mg/dL
Urine—Ketone		Strongly positive
Urine		Pathological crystals (urate, cysteine, leucine, trysine)—present
Urine—Casts, micro		One seen

Test	Low Unexpected Outcome	High Unexpected Outcome
Therapeutic Drugs		
Acetaminophen (4 h)	—	>150 µg/mL
Acetaminophen (12 h)	—	>50 µg/mL
Amikacin (peak)	—	>35 µg/mL
Amitriptyline (Nortriptyline)	—	> 450 mEq/L
Caffeine	—	>50 mg/dL
Carbamazepine	—	>20 µg/mL
Chloramphenicol (peak)	—	>50 mg/L
Clonazepam	—	>100 mEq/L
Desipramine	—	>450 mEq/L
Diazepam	—	>2.5 µg/mL
Digitoxin	—	>35 mEq/mL
Digoxin	—	>2.5 mEq/mL
Disopyramide	—	>7 mg/L
Ethosuximide	—	>200 mg/L
Flecanide	—	> 1.0 mg/L
Fluoxetine	—	> 1100 mEq/L
Gentamicin (peak)	—	> 12 mg/L
Imipramine (Desipramine)	—	> 450 mEq/L
Lidocaine	—	> 9 mg/L
Lithium	—	> 2 mEq/L
Methotrexate (high dose)	—	> 41 µg/dL
Maprotiline	—	> 1000 mEq/L
NAPA	—	> 25 mg/L
NAPA + procainamide	—	>30 mg/L
Nortriptyline	—	> 450 mEq/L
Phenobarbital	—	> 60 µg/mL
Phenytoin	—	> 40 µg/mL
Primidone	—	> 24 µg/mL
Protriptyline	—	> 450 mEq/L
Quinidine	—	> 10 µg/mL
Salicylate	—	> 700 µg/mL
Theophylline	—	> 25 µg/mL
Tobramycin (peak)	—	> 12 mg/L
Tocainide	—	12–15 µg/mL
Trazodone	—	> 3000 mEq/L
Trimipramine	—	> 450 mEq/L
Valproic acid	—	> 150 mg/L
Vancomycin (peak)	—	> 40 mg/L

Appendix D
·················

Standards for
Latex Allergy Precautions and
Diagnostic Tests and Procedures

Nursing Practice Standard

The nurse follows appropriate latex allergy precautions when caring for patients undergoing diagnostic tests and procedures.

As allergy to latex products in the health care setting becomes more common, it is necessary for agencies to institute specific protocols to maximize a latex-free environment for safety of nurse and patient and minimize risks. Reactions may vary from mild symptoms such as a slight rash to severe anaphylactic reactions—certain patients, such as those with spina bifida, are especially sensitive.

Latex Allergy Precautions to Protect the Patient

- Post appropriate signs, "Latex Allergy Precautions." Signs should be readily visible to all who care for patients; chart should also be flagged. Place patient in a private room, if possible. Schedule invasive procedures early in day if possible when latex allergen exposure is less.
- Require persons caring for latex-allergy patient to wear freshly laundered uniforms or scrubs that have not yet been exposed to other patients. Use nonlatex gloves, endotracheal tubes, suction and drainage tubes, adhesive tape, wound drains, tourniquets, temperature probe covers, and catheters for all procedures. Use latex-free blood pressure cuffs; if not available, put stockinette over patient's arm before applying cuff. Tubing can be shielded with adhesive tape if necessary. Remove rubber stoppers from vials before reconstituting medications. Do not draw medications through rubber stopper.
- Rinse syringes with sterile water or sterile saline prior to use. Remove latex ports from IV tubing and replace with stopcocks or non-latex plugs if latex-free tubing is not available.

- Keep resuscitation equipment and emergency supplies accessible at all times to be prepared for a potential severe allergy reaction.

Latex Allergy Precautions to Protect the Nurse

- Use only latex-free gloves when providing nursing procedures that require use of gloves. Avoid exposure to any latex products when providing nursing interventions.
- Encourage agency to purchase only latex-free products if at all possible.
- Wash hands thoroughly whenever involved with latex products.
- Follow all of the above listed latex allergy precautions for patients precisely to protect self and patient.

Appendix E
....

Standards for Timed Urine Specimen Collection

Nursing Practice Standard

The nurse intervenes appropriately when collecting and handling timed urine specimens, including storing in a container with specific preservative, protection of specimen from light, and refrigeration to avoid delay in test outcomes and undue patient care costs.

TEST	PRESERVATIVE	HANDLING SPECIMEN
Acid mucopoly-saccharides	20 mL Tulene	
Aldosterone	1g boric acid/ 100 mL urine	
Amylase	None	Refrig. during coll.

(cont'd.)

TEST	PRESERVATIVE	HANDLING SPECIMEN
Arsenic	None or 30 mL 6NHCl	
Cadmium	None	Refrig. during coll.
Calcium	30 mL 6NHCl	Refrig. during coll.
Catecholamines	30 mL 6NHCl	pH 1–3
Chloride	None	Refrig. during coll.
Citrate (citric acid)	30 mL 6NHCl	pH 1–3
Copper	None or 30 mL 6NHCl	Refrig. during coll.
Cortisol (free)	1.0g boric acid	Refrig. during coll.
Creatinine	None	Refrig. during coll.
Creatinine clearance	None	Refrig. during coll.
Cystine	None	Refrig. during coll.
Delta-aminolevulinic acid (ALA)	30 mL of 33% glacial acetic acid	Protect/light freeze
Electrolytes (Na,K)	None, or 1.0g boric acid	Refrigerate
Estrogens (total/ nonpregnancy or third trimester)	1.0g boric acid	Refrig. during coll.
FIGLU	12 mL Glacial acetic acid	Refrigerate
FSH/LH	1.0g boric acid	
Glucose	1.0g boric acid	
5-HIAA (serotonin)	1.0g boric acid	
Histamine	Refrigerate	
Homovanillic acid	None	Refrig. during coll.
17 Hydroxycorti- costeroids	1.0g boric acid	pH 4-7
Hydroxyproline	None	Refrig. during coll.
17 Ketogenic steroid (Porter-Silber)	1.0g boric acid	Do not refrigerate
17 Ketosteroids (total)	1.0g boric acid	Do not refrigerate
Lead	30 mL 6NHCL	Use lead-free container
Lipase	None	Refrigerate
Magnesium	None	Refrig. during coll.
Metanephrine (total)	30 mL 6NHCL	pH 1–3
Mercury	30 mL 6NHCL	pH-2 with nitric acid

TEST	PRESERVATIVE	HANDLING SPECIMEN
Oxalate	30 mL 6NHCL	pH 2–3
Phosphorous (inorganic)	None	Refrig. during coll.
Pregnanediol	1.0g boric acid	
Preganediol	1.0g boric acid	
Porphobilinogen (quantitative)	None	Refrig. during coll. protect from light
Porphyrins (uro/copro)	None (preservative added upon receipt in lab)	Protect from light
Schilling	None	Refrig. during coll. transport entire specimen to lab.
Thiocyanate	None	Refrig. during coll.
Total protein	None	Refrig. during coll.
Urea nitrogen	None	Refrigerate
Uric acid	None	Refrig. during coll.
Urobilinogen	None	Refrig. during coll.
Vanillylmandelic acid (VMA)	30 mL 6NHCL	pH 1-3; protect from light

Appendix F
....

Standards for Universal Precautions

Nursing Practice Standard

The nurse follows specific standards for universal precautions as mandated by the Occupational Safety and Health Administration (OSHA) in all health care settings to protect both self and patient.

Universal precautions protect health care workers from exposure to blood-borne pathogens and other potentially infectious materials from body fluids of all persons, including both living and dead. The Occupational Safety and Health Administration (OSHA) enforces universal precautions, a system of infectious disease control procedures, when caring for patients in all health care settings.

• • • • • • • • • • • • •

CLINICAL ALERT

- It is important for nurses to protect and always take care of themselves first. Presume that *all* patients have hepatitis B or AIDS.

• • • • • • • • • • • • •

Universal Precaution Standards and Practices for Specific Situations

Personal Protection Equipment

- Take appropriate barrier precautions when exposure of skin and mucus membranes to blood, blood droplets and other body fluids is anticipated.
- Use protective equipment devices for providing protection to eyes, face, head, extremities, air passages, and clothing. This equipment must always be used during invasive procedures.

Gloves

- Wear gloves when collecting and handling specimens, touching blood, urine, and other body fluids, mucus membranes, and/or nonintact skin of all patients.
- Wear gloves when handling items or surfaces soiled with blood, urine, or body fluids; for performing venipuncture or other vascular access procedures; and for all invasive procedures.
- Mandate wearing gloves when the nurse's skin is cut, abraded, chapped or when the nurse is involved in examining patient's oropharynx, Gl or GU tract, nonintact or abraded skin, active bleeding wounds, or when cleaning specimen containers involving body fluids or decontaminating procedures.

Gowns, Masks and Eye Protection

- Require wearing gowns, aprons, and/or lab coats to cover all exposed skin whenever there is potential of splashing on clothing

- Wear mask and goggles (prescription glasses) when contamination of eye, nose, or mouth from sepsis is most likely to occur.
- Not required for routine nursing care in situations where contamination from blood, urine, or body fluids is not likely to occur.
- Provide mouth-to-mouth emergency resuscitation equipment in strategic locations in all clinical settings.

Disposal of Medical Wastes

- Take precautions to prevent injuries caused by needles, scalpels, other sharp instruments or devices during and after procedures, and when disposing of used needles.
- Dispose of all sharp instruments in puncture-resistant containers. Do not recap, bend, break by hand, or remove needles for disposable syringes.
- Place and transport specimen in leak-proof receptacles with solid, tight-fitting covers. Before transport, contaminated materials are decontaminated or placed in a tightly sealed bag or marked with a "biohazard" tag.

Placement of Warning Tags and Signs

- Use warning tags to prevent accidental injury or illness to nurses who are exposed to equipment or procedures that are hazardous, unexpected or unusual .
- Require warning tags to contain a *signal word* or symbol, such as "Biohazard," or "Biochemical Material" with the major message such as, "Blood Banking Specimen Inside."

General Environmental Cautions

- Wash hands immediately after removing gloves.
- Wash hands and other skin surfaces immediately and thoroughly if contaminated with blood or other body fluids.
- Consider saliva potentially infectious, even though it has not been implicated in HIV transmission.
- Transmission of AIDS disease is possible from stool specimens, especially if there is a possibility of blood existing in the stool.

In Case of HIV or Hepatitis B HBV Exposure:

- Identify, obtain consent, and test source of exposure (patients with AIDS or Hepatitis B infection). If patient refuses consent or outcome is positive, the nurse *must* receive HIV antibody testing immediately.

- Advise HIV negative nurses to seek medical evaluation of any acute febrile illness within 12 weeks of exposure to AIDS and retest 6–12 weeks, and 6 months after exposure.

References
• • • • • • • • • • • • • • •

Anderson, S. (1990, August). ABGs: Six easy steps to interpreting blood gases. *American Journal of Nursing*, *90*(8): 42–45.

Avey, M. A. (1993, September). TB skin testing: How to do it right. *American Journal of Nursing*, *93*(9): 42–44.

Baum, S. et al. (1993). *Atlas of nuclear medicine imaging*, 2nd ed. Norwalk, CT: Appleton and Lange.

Blevins, S. J. & Benson, S. (1992, October). A better way to get kids through scans. *RN*, *55* (10): 40–45.

Bowles, K. & Lynch, M. (1992, July). These products and procedures prevent needle sticks. *RN*, *55*(7): 42–45.

Brandt, B. (1990, January–February). Nursing protocol for the patient with neutropenia. *Oncology Nursing Forum*, *17*(1 suppl.): 10.

Buffington, S. (1991, December). How much do you know about laboratory studies? *Nursing 91*, *21*(12): 46–49.

Cheney, A. M. & Maquindang, M. L. (1993, April). Patient teaching for x-ray and other diagnostics: Transesophageal echocardiogram. *RN*, *56*(4): 54–56.

Cherniack, R. M. (Ed.). (1992). *Pulmonary function testing*, 5th ed. Philadelphia: W. B. Saunders Company.

Cooper, C. (1993, August). What color is that urine specimen? *American Journal of Nursing*, *93*(8): 37.

Cuzzell, J. Z. (1993, May). The right way to culture a wound. *American Journal of Nursing*, *93*(5): 48–50.

Fischbach, F. T. (1992). *A manual of laboratory and diagnostic tests*. 4th ed. Philadelphia: J.B. Lippincott Company.

Fischbach, F. T. (1991). *Documenting care—Communication, the nursing process and documentation standards*. Philadelphia: F.A. Davis Company.

Fritsch, D. E. & Pilat, D. M. F. (1993, August). Exposing latex allergies. *Nursing 1993, 23*(8): 46–48.

Gawlikowski, J. (1992, March). White cells at war. *American Journal of Nursing, 92*(3): 44–51.

Geissler, E. M. (1991, April). Transcultural nursing and nursing diagnosis. *Nursing and Health Care, 12*(4): 190–203.

Hochrein, M. & Sohl, L. (1992, December). Heart smart: A guide to cardiac tests. *American Journal of Nursing, 92*(12): 22–25.

Huddleston, V. B. (1991, September). Multisystem organ failure: What you need to know. *Nursing '91, 21*(9): 34–43.

Jordon, C. D. et al. (1992, September 3). Normal reference values. *New England Journal of Medicine, 327*(10): 718–724.

Kestel, F. (1993, March). Using blood glucose meters: What you and your patient need to know, Part I. *Nursing '93, 23*(3): 34–38. Part II. *Nursing '93, 23*(4): 50–53. Part III. *Nursing '93, 23*(5): 51–55.

Laraen, S. A. et al. (1990). *A manual of tests for syphilis*, 8th ed. Washington, D. C.: American Public Health Association.

Lavin, J. & Haidorfer, C. (1993, September). Anergy testing—A vital weapon. *RN, 56*(9): 31–32.

Leavelle, D. (Ed.) (1992). *Mayo Medical Laboratories, interpretive handbook*, Rochester, MN.

Martin, J. P. (1991, February). Transrectal ultrasound: A new screening tool for prostate cancer. *American Journal of Nursing, 91*(2): 69.

Marx, J. F. (1993, January). Viral hepatitis: Unscrambling the alphabet. *Nursing '93, 23*(1): 34–42.

McDonagh, A. (1991, February). Getting your patient ready for a nuclear medicine scan. *Nursing '91, 21*(2): 53–57.

Merrich, P. A., Case, B. J. et al. (1991, January). Care of pediatric patients sedated with pentobarbital sodium in MRI. *Pediatric Nursing, 17*(1): 35.

Millam, D. A. (1993, July). How to teach good venipuncture technique. *American Journal of Nursing, 93*(7): 38–41.

Mims, B. C. (1991, March). Interpreting ABGs. *RN, 54*(3): 42–47.

Monroe, D. (1991, February). Patient teaching for x-ray and other diagnostics (cardiac catheterization). *RN, 54*(2): 44–46.

National Blood Resource Education Program's Nursing Education Work Group. (1991, June). Transfusion Nursing: Trends and Practice for the 90s (4 part article). *American Journal of Nursing, 91*(6): 42–56.

Olbrych, D. D. (1993, January). Interpreting C. P. K. and L. D. H. results. *Nursing '93, 23*(1): 48–49.

Pinner, J. (1991, March). Patient teaching for x-ray and other diagnostic (stress tests). *RN, 54*(3): 32–36.

Renkes, J. (1993, June). G. I. endoscopy: Managing the full scope of care. *Nursing '93, 23*(6): 50–55.

Schultz, S. J., Foley, C. R. & Gordon, D. G. (1991, September). Preparing your patient for a cardiac P.E.T. scan. *Nursing '91, 21*(9): 63–64.

Sergi, N. A. (1991, March). When your patient need a stress test. *RN, 54*(3): 26–31.

Sieh, A. & Brentin, L. (1993, March). A little light makes venipuncture easier. *RN, 56*(3): 40–43.

Solomon, J. (1992, May). Taking the EKG one step further. *RN, 55*(5): 56–60.

Stiesmeyer, J. K. (1993, August). A four-step approach to pulmonary assessment. *American Journal of Nursing, 93*(8): 22–28.

Trustem, A. (1991, August). When to suspect ectopic pregnancy. *RN, 54*(8): 22–25.

Wallach, J. (1992). *Interpretation of diagnostic tests. Synopsis of laboratory medicine*, 5th ed. Boston: Little, Brown & Co.

Weikert, C. J. (1993, October). New eye into the heart (position emission tomography). *RN, 56*(10): 36–39.

Wilkinson, M. (1990, Fall). Nursing implications after endoscopic retrograde cholangiopancreatograph. *Gastroenterology Nursing, 13*(2): 105–109.

Yarnell, R. P. & Craig, M. P. (1991, July). Detecting hypomagnesemia: The most overlooked electrolyte imbalance. *Nursing '91, 21*(7): 55–57.

Index

· · · · · · · · · ·

Page numbers followed by a t indicate table; numbers followed by
an f indicate figure.